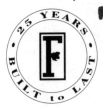

SOLVING PROSTATE PROBLEMS

Answers and Advice
from a Leading Expert

MARTIN K. GELBARD, M.D.
& WILLIAM BENTLEY

A FIRESIDE BOOK
Published by Simon & Schuster
New York   London   Toronto   Sydney   Tokyo   Singapore

FIRESIDE
Rockefeller Center
1230 Avenue of the Americas
New York, New York 10020

FIRESIDE and colophon are registered trademarks of Simon & Schuster Inc.

Designed by Irving Perkins Associates
Illustrations by Martin K. Gelbard, M.D.
Manufactured in the United States of America

1   3   5   7   9   10   8   6   4   2

Library of Congress Cataloging-in-Publication Data

Gelbard, Martin K.
Solving prostate problems : answers and advice from a leading
expert / by Martin K. Gelbard & William Bentley.
p.   cm.
''A Fireside book.''
Includes index.
1. Prostate—Diseases—Popular works.   I. Bentley, William.
II. Title.
RC899.G44   1995
616.6′5—dc20   94-26400
                                                                         CIP

ISBN: 0-671-88465-4

CONTENTS

INTRODUCTION

Solving Prostate Problems began as an information booklet for patients and their families; it was written for both men and women. True, only men have a prostate, but the worry caused by its disorders affects both men and women. The goal of this book is to dispel the fear and anxiety produced by problems in this often misunderstood male "Achilles' heel."

The prostate gland draws little attention until later in life, but the lessons learned from medical research and patient care can be helpful at any age. By reviewing the function (and malfunction) of this organ, and answering the basic questions that pop up in the minds of patients, we hope to relieve many common concerns. "Feeling good about yourself" may be a secondary effect of increased understanding, but our primary effort has been to go much deeper than mere reassurance. Contemporary research is surveyed and summarized in a style containing enough scientific fact to be authoritative, yet broad enough in example and illustration to remain easily accessible to the nonmedical reader.

This is not a science text, but most of the book stays within the confines of what is generally considered scientific knowledge. We occasionally venture beyond these boundaries to examine traditional, herbal, or folk remedies and some of the popular mythology that surrounds the prostate gland.

Science is a method of building understanding out of observation, not a collection of unchanging facts. If ideas about the prostate and medical practice change from year to year, it is more a reflection of this process than of the fickle nature of doctors. Scientific knowledge is an ever-enlarging structure, which despite its sparkle and scope is never completed. Science cannot translate nature into an ultimate plan and parts list; nature refuses complete categorization, retaining her wildness even under the closest scrutiny.

Like so much in medicine, we can't get started without a disclaimer: this book is not intended to replace medical care. Its purpose is to provide information and assistance in getting the most out of a doctor's visit—if that is necessary. In the sections that follow, a sampling of what has been learned about the prostate, both in health and in disease, is presented. Its structure and normal function are described, and factors identified that lead to bothersome symptoms or disorders. Nutrition and other health maintenance programs or preventive measures will also be discussed, as well as the effects of prostate problems on sexual function.

To understand the symptoms produced by the prostate, we digress into human plumbing as a basis for discussing urinary and sexual difficulties. Current technology has produced a number of new and interesting means to measure and study these problems. Descriptions of these methods, the information they provide, and the science behind them will increase the reader's understanding of specific disorders. Infections, infertility, sexual dysfunction, benign prostatic enlargement, and cancer are reviewed in depth. Ways to keep the prostate healthy are outlined, as well as what can be done in the event of problems.

<figure>FIGURE 1-1

Overall Anatomy</figure>

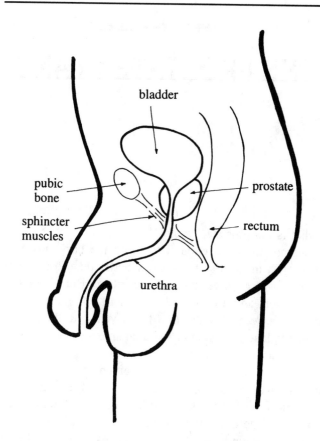

WHERE IS THE PROSTATE?

In order to understand where the prostate is situated and how it functions within the urinary and reproductive tracts, we need to briefly cover the overall "layout" of a man's internal plumbing.

The urethra serves two systems. The first is the system for waste removal and the maintenance of the body's internal fluid balance: the *kidneys, ureters, bladder,* and *urethra.* The second system is

Chapter 1

THE PROSTATE GLAND

"Just what is the prostate, Doctor?"

My patients are good enough to bring me back down to earth when I get lost in details. They know better than to ask where the prostate is, for fear I'll get out a rubber glove. But it's nevertheless a good question, and a proper place to start.

Only men have a prostate. In a thirty-year-old, the prostate is a walnut-sized gland that weighs less than an ounce and surrounds the *urethra* (urinary channel).

The *prostatic urethra* is the name given to that section of the delicate tube which traverses the prostate, discharging urine to the outside world when the bladder is full. I mention "young men" and "walnut-sized" here, for the prostate tends to enlarge as men age. The prostate surrounds the urethra much like a donut. In fact, the prostate is actually part of the urethra—it develops from the urethra itself.

The male lower urinary tract must alternate between its most frequent role as plumbing for the excretion of urine and its occasional role as a delivery system for semen during the act of ejaculation. Women are fortunate enough to have independent duct systems for urinary excretion and reproduction, whereas men must put extra wear and tear on their plumbing because of this time-sharing arrangement.

FIGURE 1-2
The Urethra and Ejaculatory Ducts

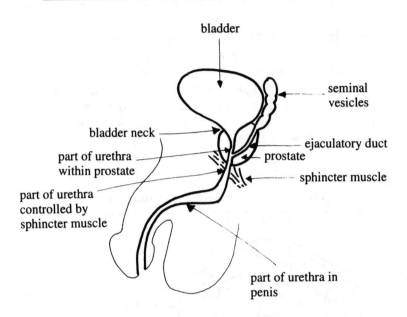

made up of the structures responsible for reproduction: the *testes* and their duct systems, the prostate, and the *seminal vesicles.* Because the prostate is part of the urethra, it belongs to both of these systems.

The urethra is a tube for conducting urine from the bladder to the outside world. In men it is about 8 inches long, with the upper 1½ inches traversing the prostate. The urethra then traverses the muscular floor of the pelvis. This ¼- to ½-inch segment constitutes the *sphincter,* or valve of the urinary tract that can be controlled by will. The remaining 6 inches of urethra runs from the perineum (the area where the back side of the scrotal sack attaches to the body) out to the opening at the end of the penis.

The upper end of the urethra meets the bladder at the upper margin of the prostate, a region called the *bladder neck,* or bladder outlet. Within the prostate a main tributary to the urethra enters, carrying (during ejaculation) sperm from the testicles, and additional fluids from accessory glands called the seminal vesicles. The point within the prostate where the ejaculatory ducts join the urethra forms the final merging of a man's urinary and reproductive systems.

The prostate sits within the *pelvis,* which is a bone (actually a fused or connected set of bones) that contains the lower abdominal organs and surrounds the lower ends of both the intestinal and urinary tracts. Because of this, the rectum is immediately adjacent to the prostate, just behind it. Immediately in front of the prostate is the pubic bone, an important anatomical reference point and the forward-most point of the pelvis.

FIGURE 1-3
The Pelvis, Lower Back, and Urinary Tract

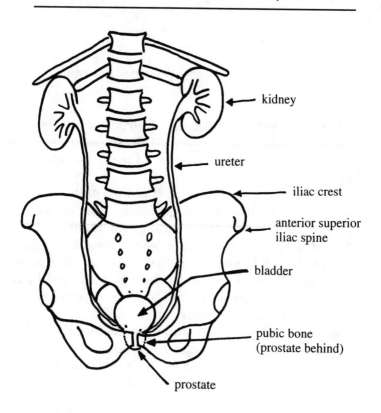

kidney

ureter

iliac crest

anterior superior iliac spine

bladder

pubic bone
(prostate behind)

prostate

The bones of the pelvis enclose the prostate, the bladder, and part of the urethra. If you stand with your hands on your hips, fingers pointing forward, your index fingers will touch the prominent points of bone on either side of the front of the abdomen. These points are called the *anterior superior iliac spines* and are an important landmark for surgeons and anatomists. The highest point of the pelvis on either side (under your thumbs) is called the *iliac crest*. Now, if you feel straight down from the belly button, you come to the lower end of the muscular wall of the abdomen, where it attaches to the pubic bone. This bony landmark can be felt at the extreme lower end of the abdomen, beneath the skin that bears pubic hair. It lies immediately in front of the prostate and contains cartilage that connects the right and left halves of the pelvis.

HOW DOES THE PROSTATE FORM?

During the third to fourth month of fetal development, the male embryo begins to develop a series of outgrowths or outpouchings from the upper end of the urethra, just below where the urethra joins the bladder. These outgrowths gradually push outward and enlarge into the surrounding connective tissue. Their multiplication and enlargement causes a segment of the upper urethra to be surrounded by a collection of microscopic chambers that empty into the urinary channel itself.

In adult life, these chambers will produce the proteins, sugars, fats, and other components of semen, specifically the milky fluid that helps transport and protect sperm through the penis during ejaculation. While the testicle is responsible for generating sperm cells, the job of giving them something to swim in, and of providing for their metabolic needs, falls in part to the prostate gland.

When the baby boy is born, the prostate is nothing more than a slightly thickened part of the upper urethra. Beginning with the onset of puberty (about ten to twelve years of age), the cells lining these outpouchings multiply, enlarging the little chambers. In addition to this, the connective and muscular tissues that were initially penetrated by the growth of these buds enlarge. By the time a young

FIGURE 1-4
Formation of the Prostate

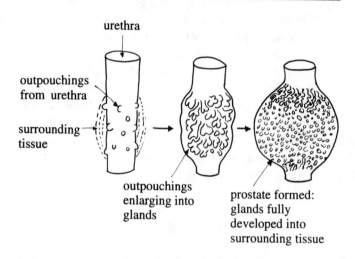

urethra

outpouchings
from urethra

surrounding
tissue

outpouchings
enlarging into
glands

prostate formed:
glands fully
developed into
surrounding tissue

young man completes puberty and matures sexually, the prostate has
doubled in weight. In the adult, the prostate weighs approximately
20 grams. By the time a man reaches the age of thirty or forty, these
gland chambers undergo more expansion, which causes them to be
infolded. Imagine that an overzealous paperhanger tries to hang five
or ten times too much wallpaper in a small room, in a single layer.
He would have to fold and wrinkle the paper off the walls out into
the room until the room begins to fill up with folds of protruding
wallpaper. This infolding of the cells lining the gland chambers
stops by age forty or fifty.

Glandular tissue within the prostate is arranged in a specific way.
Doctors studying prostate anatomy have divided the prostate into
different regions, or "zones," because it helps them understand how
and why problems may arise. Immediately next to the urethra is a
small inner region of glandular chambers called the *transition zone.*
This is surrounded by a large shell of glandular tissue called the
peripheral zone. Adjacent to this is the *central zone,* which surrounds the ejaculatory ducts, entering the prostate from the reproductive tract.

After the glandular infolding, the normal development of the prostate is complete. In the years that follow, abnormal growth of the prostate, both benign and malignant, may lead to symptoms or illness. Patterns of abnormal growth conform to the different anatomical zones of the prostate.

In general, cancers form in the peripheral zone of the prostate, whereas benign prostatic hypertrophy originates in the transitional zone. If the cells within the transitional zone multiply and enlarge dramatically, they push outward and stretch the peripheral zone into a thin shell.

Surgery is detailed in chapter 6, but this is a good time to point out that removal of the prostate to relieve blockage for benign enlargement does not remove the risk of cancer. "Doc," patients say, "you took my prostate out—how can I still get cancer?"

Surgery for benign enlargement removes the obstructing inner transitional zone, leaving the peripheral zone like a shell or a rind on the outside. Since cancers tend to form in the peripheral zone, it is still possible that the disease will develop.

In examining the formation of the prostate, we should recognize

FIGURE 1-5
Zones of the Prostate

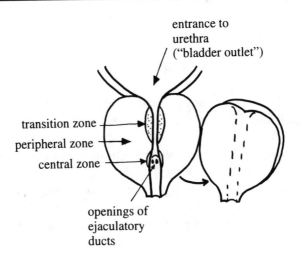

entrance to
urethra
("bladder outlet")

transition zone

peripheral zone

central zone

openings of
ejaculatory
ducts

Figure 1-6
Transitional Zone Overgrowth—BPH

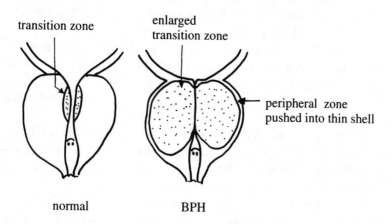

that this organ is partly muscle and supporting tissue, and partly cells that line glandular chambers and secrete substances into the seminal fluid. In the adult, about 30 percent by weight of the prostate is muscle and connective tissue, and the remaining 70 percent is secretory cells that line the glandular chambers. These two components—muscle and glandular cells—become important in the treatment of prostate enlargement with drugs, which will be discussed in chapter 5.

THE PATH OF THE SPERM CELL

The secretions of the prostate gland supply essential materials to the sperm cells that allow them to continue their high-energy activities even after they have left a man's body. Sperm cells come into existence when cells lining the testicle divide. In the process of splitting off from these "mother" cells, sperm cells receive one-half of the genetic material that is present within the human cell. When they meet up with an egg cell containing the other half, fertilization may occur. For this to happen, the sperm cell must get from the testicle to the outside world by transversing the *epididymis,* a coiled

duct along the back of the testicle that is involved in sperm maturation. This duct receives the output of the sperm-generating ducts
within the testicle and then gives way to the *vas deferens*. This
muscular tube carries the sperm cell up into the groin, around the
back of the bladder, and into the prostate. The sperm are temporarily
stored in the dilated end of the vas deferens until they enter the
urethra within the prostate at the time of ejaculation.

Where Do Sperm Enter the Urinary Tract?

When you look at a side view of the prostate, you can see that it is
the junction of two channels, or a Y connection: the urinary channel,

FIGURE 1-7
Pathway Taken by Sperm

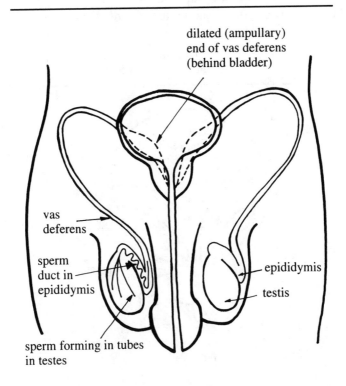

dilated (ampullary)
end of vas deferens
(behind bladder)

vas
deferens

sperm
duct in
epididymis

epididymis

testis

sperm forming in tubes
in testes

or urethra, on one side, and the reproductive channel, or ejaculatory ducts, on the other.

The ejaculatory ducts are the passageways for sperm to enter the urethra during ejaculation. During this process, the sperm become mixed with the secretions of the seminal vesicles and prostate gland. The seminal vesicles are thin muscular pouches about 2 inches long and ½ inch wide that lie along the back of the bladder, just above the prostate. They have an infolded or convoluted lining that contributes a sticky substance to semen. Each seminal vesicle holds a little less than a teaspoonful of fluid.

The vas deferens is the tube that is cut during a vasectomy. It is a firm round cord about as big as a piece of spaghetti and runs from the testicle into the groin. When the vas deferens approaches the prostate, it becomes slightly dilated and is called the *ampullary vas.* This dilated end of the vas deferens stores up the sperm, which are subsequently discharged by the muscular contractions of its walls into the ejaculatory ducts and urethra during ejaculation.

FIGURE 1-8
The Back of the Bladder

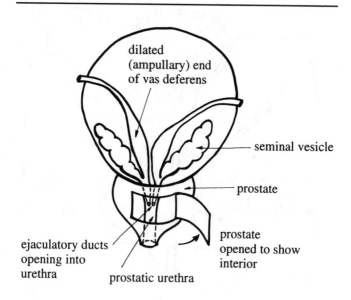

dilated
(ampullary) end
of vas deferens

seminal vesicle

prostate

ejaculatory ducts
opening into
urethra

prostate
opened to show
interior

prostatic urethra

THE UPPER URINARY TRACT

The upper part of the urinary tract is composed of the kidneys and ureters, which lie higher in the trunk along the inner wall of the back (see figure 1–3). While standing with hands on your hips and your thumbs pointing back, slide your hands upward along your sides until your index fingers first touch your ribs. At this position, the kidneys are just under your thumbs. The kidney is a paired, fist-sized organ that is highly specialized for the filtration of waste products from the blood and serves a critical function in keeping the chemical makeup of our internal fluids constant. In addition, it has a role in metabolism and in creating a hormonal signal for red blood cell production. It is also a key component in regulating blood pressure.

By an effective system of filtration followed by reabsorption of the filtered fluid, the kidney processes about two hundred quarts of blood every day, resulting in the production of a few pints of urine.

THE PATH OF A DROP OF URINE

Blood pumping through the kidney enters the smaller and smaller vessels and is finally channeled into a tangle of tiny capillaries called a *glomerulus,* one of many contained in the kidney. This little tuft of capillaries is cupped in the end of a long tube, the *nephron.* When a drop of blood is filtered out of the glomerulus and enters the nephron, it contains vital ingredients as well as waste products. As the drop passes down the nephron the desired ingredients are reabsorbed back into the bloodstream, leaving a drop that contains mostly unwanted waste products. The output of all the nephrons in the kidney finally collects in the *renal pelvis,* a small funnel in the center of the kidney that empties into a specialized tube, the ureter.

Urine does not freely move down the ureters by gravity but must be gently propelled by *peristalsis,* a coordinated squeezing action of the ureters' wall. When we discuss urinary tract obstruction by the prostate, we will see how this can change. You cannot feel your ureteral peristalsis unless it becomes abnormally powerful, as occurs when the body is attempting to expel a kidney stone.

WHERE IS THE BLADDER?

The *bladder* is a hollow muscular container for the storage and periodic expulsion of urine. In a newborn it lies within the lower abdomen, but in an adult it is well down within the bones of the pelvis. It is behind and slightly above the pubic bone when full and is separated from the rectum behind it by the paired seminal vesicles. Urine will not flow out of the bladder and into the toilet by the force of gravity alone. The bladder must actively work and contract to expel urine. For it to work effectively in emptying urine, its muscle, which is controlled by nerve impulses, must contract. The bladder also works as a storage organ, allowing urine to collect without causing discomfort. To do this, it must be able to fill with little increase in muscle tension.

WHAT IS A GLAND?

A gland is an organ specialized for secretion. Glands come in two varieties: those that secrete products into the bloodstream (*endocrine glands,* such as the thyroid) and those whose secretion products are delivered into a special duct system for direct delivery into an organ (*exocrine glands,* such as the salivary glands). The prostate is an exocrine gland that secrets constituents of semen.

CELLS

Living structures are built up of microscopic units called *cells.* Cells contain a central package, the *nucleus,* which has all the information necessary to form and operate our marvelous bodily structure. This information is contained in the arrangement of special molecules, deoxyribonucleic acid (*DNA*), which form the chromosomes. Surrounding the nucleus is the outer part of the cell, which contains all of the structures and enzymes necessary to conduct its daily chemical business.

HUMAN STRUCTURE: ONE BLUEPRINT, MANY DIFFERENT CELLS

In a gland, the secretion of substances begins in its constituent cells. Each gland produces a limited and customized output. The cells in a man's prostate contain genetic information identical with that found in every other one of his cells, yet they produce a limited variety of proteins. Even though this genetic information, a blueprint for manufacturing every protein made by the body, is identical in all cells, cells differ considerably in what portion of the blueprint they use, based on their intended specialization. For example, muscle cells contain different proteins than fat cells. Different collections of cells, or living tissues, are composed of cells that are using only a limited part of their genetic programming. The prostate is a collection of cells that have individualized their programming to produce the proteins and nutrients necessary for the well-being and normal function of sperm cells

SECRETION IN THE PROSTATE GLAND

In the prostate, materials released from an individual cell are channeled into the reproductive tract in an organized way. Separate cells are arranged next to one another until they form little chambers with a single passageway leading out. Imagine a grapevine in reverse— instead of the grapes being nourished by the earth, the fruit feeds the ground by sending materials through the stems into the branches and down the main trunk. In fact, the medical term for the primary chamber in a secretory gland is *alveolus,* which comes from the Greek word for grape.

These tributary ducts coming from groups of secretory glands gradually run together and then empty into a central region in the prostatic urethra. During ejaculation, their secretions are mixed with

FIGURE 1-9
Gland Structure

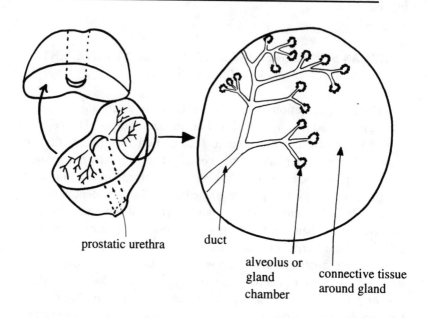

prostatic urethra   duct

alveolus or
gland   connective tissue
chamber   around gland

the spermatozoa and secretion of the seminal vesicles, which enter into the same region of the urethra through two channels, the *ejaculatory ducts.*

A very low level of prostate secretion occurs steadily. In part, this may have a protective effect against infections intruding on the lower urinary tract. During ejaculation, secretion is increased. The delivery of sperm from the terminal vas deferens and secretions of the seminal vesicles, prostate, and other minor urethral glands is coordinated by specific neurological input.

NERVE CONTROL IN THE PROSTATE

Ejaculation is a neurological phenomenon coordinated by the sympathetic nervous system, one of the "automatic control" networks of nerves affecting bodily function that is not controlled by will-power. This process is separate from that of erection. Following operations that disturb certain regions of the sympathetic nervous system, a man may lose his ability to ejaculate, although erection and some sensation of climax are preserved. Nerves have been traced to muscle-containing regions within the prostate gland, and around the seminal vesicles. These muscles contract, squeezing out secretions during ejaculation. The muscle cells lining the upper half of the prostatic urethra respond to a special type of nerve stimulation, characterized by what are termed *alpha-adrenergic receptors.* These are chemical communication links or molecular sites on cells that respond to certain substances. Drugs that block these receptors prevent muscle contraction from narrowing the urethral channel in this area, and improve urinary flow in men with symptoms of blockage due to benign prostatic enlargement.

WHAT DO PROSTATE AND SEMINAL VESICLE SECRETIONS CONTAIN?

Semen is unique among bodily fluids in that it contains high concentrations of materials that are found in only trace amounts or not at all in other bodily fluids. The average amount of fluid passed during ejaculation is about three milliliters. Of this, one and a half to two milliliters come from the seminal vesicles and one-half milliliter from the prostate. A small additional amount comes from other glands of the urethra. The testicle and epididymis contribute less than 1 percent to the volume of ejaculation, including the volume of the sperm cells themselves.

The prostate gland has the highest level of zinc of any organ and contributes high concentrations of zinc to semen, which probably has an antibacterial effect. However, altering the dietary intake of zinc does not change the zinc content of semen. Fructose, a sugar secreted by the seminal vesicles, serves as a fuel supply or energy source for the sperm cells. The seminal vesicles produce high levels of *prostaglandins,* chemicals that affect sperm movement and muscular activity within male and female genital tracts. They have been shown to affect vaginal and cervical secretions as well as the rate of sperm transport through the female genital tract.

The prostate and its secretions also contain higher levels of citric acid than occur elsewhere in the body, though the function of citric acid in semen is not known. The prostate is also active in secreting fats—cholesterol and lipids—into semen. Some researchers believe that these compounds may protect the sperm against environmental or temperature shock.

PROSTATE-SPECIFIC ANTIGEN (PSA)

Many proteins are secreted by the prostate. One of these, *gamma-seminoprotein*, is involved in the liquefaction of semen. This protein has attained critical diagnostic importance in the last five years or so as a useful test for evaluating prostate cancer. Measurement of gamma-seminoprotein activity in the blood gives a number known as the *PSA*, or *prostate-specific antigen* value. The use of this measurement is described in chapters 3 and 6.

WHAT CONTROLS PROSTATE GROWTH?

Understanding prostate growth is particularly important as we look at prostate disorders, including prostate cancer. Cells multiply within the gland chambers, and this process must be regulated. Cells lining the glands are actively involved in the metabolic processes of synthesis and secretion and are subject to the stresses and wear of continued activity. They die and are sloughed into the gland, and to take their place, other cells divide and multiply. To keep the proper balance required for continued secretion, there must be sensitive control over cell death and cell proliferation.

We are beginning to learn about the regulation of this process, although much of it remains a mystery. Errors or malfunctions in the regulation of cell growth and division are probably very close to the actual cause of cancer.

FIGURE 1-10
Cellular Growth and Death Within the Gland

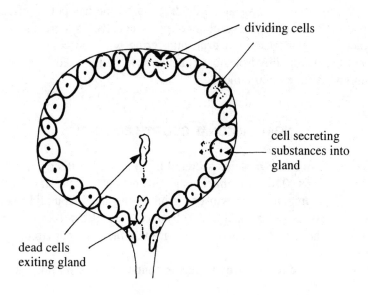

dividing cells

cell secreting
substances into
gland

dead cells
exiting gland

TESTOSTERONE

Many different systems of control affect prostatic growth; including hormonal signals sent through the bloodstream from other areas. The male sex hormone, *testosterone,* is manufactured primarily in the testes, although the adrenal gland produces a small amount. This hormone is responsible for the growth of the prostate at puberty, and its presence is required in the adult for maintenance of prostate size and secretory capacity. Withdrawal of testosterone by castration results in the loss of about 90 percent of prostate gland lining cells and a loss of about 40 percent of the supportive or connective tissue cells within the prostate. For this reason, either castration or some form of hormone removal has long been used successfully to shrink prostate tumors in patients with prostate cancer.

Testosterone itself is not directly responsible for interacting with the metabolic machinery within the prostate cell. Once testosterone has entered the prostate cell, it must be converted to a compound called *dihydrotestosterone* by the action of *5-alpha reductase,* an enzyme within the prostate. Dihydrotestosterone has potent effects upon the growth and metabolism of prostate cells. This process is of practical importance, as a drug interfering with the conversion of testosterone to dihydrotestosterone is now being used to reverse benign prostate enlargement.

NONHORMONAL GROWTH CONTROL

Growth factors are proteins secreted by other cells directly into the body's fluids. These chemical signals may affect prostate cells, either by stimulating growth or by inhibiting it. Surrounding connective tissues or extracellular substances can also affect prostate cells or their response to protein growth factors and circulating hormones.

Such interaction or growth factor contact occurs initially at the

FIGURE 1-11
Control of Cell Growth

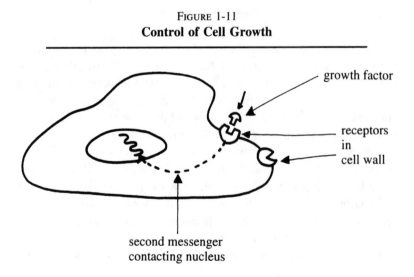

growth factor

receptors
in
cell wall

second messenger
contacting nucleus

outer wall, or cell membrane, of the prostate cell. To carry this message from the cell membrane into the nucleus, where cell division and growth begin, there is a second messenger system. Much current evidence suggests that alterations in this messenger system are closely related to the events initiating cancer.

Chapter 2

====

SYMPTOMS OF PROSTATE PROBLEMS

You're standing in a men's room at a packed stadium, trying to relieve yourself quickly into a large trough while fifteen or twenty of your fellow spectators are doing the same. Never mind that half of these men have just swilled copious amounts of beer or that five or six men are lined up behind you squirming, tapping their toes, waiting . . .

CAN NORMAL MEN HAVE TROUBLE URINATING?

Yes, but this simple answer immediately calls to mind another, more bothersome question: when do symptoms originating in the urinary tract signal trouble? The answer to this is not so simple. Even after reviewing the anatomy and normal function of a man's plumbing, we still do not have the perspective necessary to separate nuisance complaints from warnings about impending disaster. This is one of the more refined skills used by experienced doctors and, in the final analysis, requires that level of expertise. This chapter will not provide immediate medical training. By reviewing the symptoms, tests, and examinations used to evaluate patients suspected of urinary tract malfunction, we hope to help allay the anxiety associated with common symptoms, and improve communication between you and your doctor should testing be necessary.

PROBLEMS WITH URINATION

The prostate does not merely surround or encircle the urethra. As we discussed, it arises from the upper urethra during embryonic growth. Because of this, the prostate gland is really part of the urethra. The urinary channel is a tube, or duct, with about the same diameter as a pencil. Although we frequently refer to this tube as "plumbing," its behavior and ability to conduct the flow of urine is quite different from that of a rigid pipe. Particularly in the upper, or prostatic, urethra, flexibility, elasticity, and distensibility are important in allowing the free flow of urine.

When abnormalities in this section of the plumbing occur, the normal effortless relief of emptying the bladder can turn into an ordeal of waiting, coaxing, straining, and dribbling.

Figure 2-1
Changes in Upper Urethra with Urination

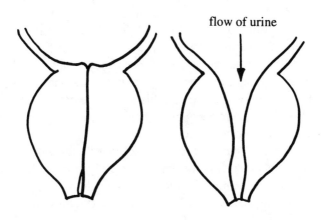

flow of urine

Frequency

Under normal conditions of fluid intake and perspiration, the kidneys produce about 30 to 50 milliliters (6 to 8 tablespoons) of urine per hour. The bladder capacity in most men averages 250 to 300 milliliters, which means that one should be able to go four to five hours between pit stops in the restroom. The average man voids five to six times every twenty-four hours. Of course, more frequent urination may be caused by increased fluid intake or by *diuretics* (substances that promote the excretion of urine). Diabetes is a classic example of this condition, as a loss of sugar in the urine results in secondary fluid loss and increased urinary output. Cold weather causes constriction of peripheral, or superficial, blood vessels, to reduce the body's heat loss. This effectively reduces the space for circulating blood, which results in the kidney's adjusting to the situation accordingly. It reabsorbs less of the filtered blood, increasing urinary excretion and resulting in urinary frequency. Cold also has an effect on the bladder muscle, making it less flexible and less able to accommodate amounts of urine without pulling too tight and feeling full.

"A weak bladder," or *frequency,* is one of the most common urinary symptoms. In addition to any causes of increased kidney output, conditions that reduce the storage capacity of the bladder will bring about increased frequency of urination. The muscle of the bladder wall is normally very soft and flexible, expanding easily as the bladder fills up. If the bladder wall loses this flexibility and becomes stiffer for any reason, frequency may result.

Infections and other disorders such as bladder stones and bladder cancer also cause irritation of the bladder wall, making storage of urine difficult and increasing frequency. Infections adjacent to the bladder can cause urinary frequency as well.

Ineffective bladder emptying can also contribute to the problem. Normally, the bladder should empty completely after voiding. When the bladder becomes gradually blocked, as can happen with prostate enlargement, the bladder can lose its ability to empty completely.

FIGURE 2-2
Bladder Wall Behavior

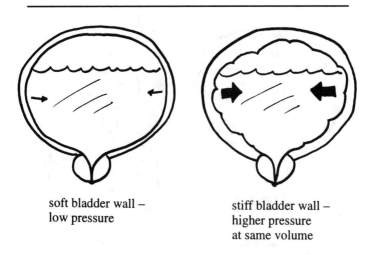

soft bladder wall –
low pressure

stiff bladder wall –
higher pressure
at same volume

This results in frequent urination of small amounts—"taking the top off" when the bladder gets full, but never completely emptying it.

Getting up to urinate too many times during the night is a classic symptom of prostate problems. Like frequency, it can have many causes, but in chronic, or long-standing, blockage of the bladder due to prostate enlargement, it is caused by increased stiffness of the bladder wall. This is a result of the body's attempt to overcome the blockage by increasing the muscularity of the bladder. As the muscle of the bladder grows stronger and thicker, pushing harder against the blockage, it becomes less flexible. This makes efficient voiding of nightly urine production more difficult.

Normally a person gets up no more than twice a night to urinate. An increase in this average can be due to heart disease, when weakness of the heart as a pump allows fluid to collect in the body's tissues during the day. When our posture changes from upright to recumbent at night, physical factors increase the reabsorption of this fluid into the bloodstream. This increases blood flow to the kidney, urine output, and urinary frequency.

Age-related changes in kidney function may also contribute to

FIGURE 2-3
Bladder Emptying

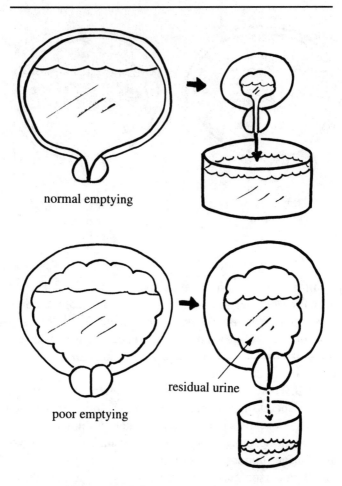

nighttime voiding. The kidney can usually get rid of waste products with a minimal loss of water by making very concentrated urine. Say you've had a margarita with salt on the glass, and you're dehydrated—your system is low on water but doesn't need the salt. Since you can't excrete the salt in granulated form, you have to use some of the water your body needs to flush out the salt. The older you get, the more water is required to do this.

FIGURE 2-4
Concentrating Ability

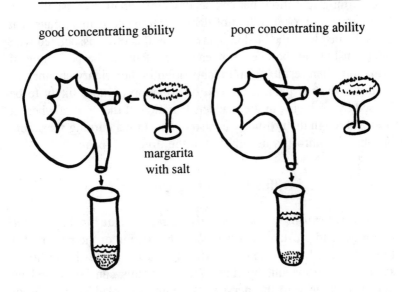

good concentrating ability   poor concentrating ability

margarita
with salt

Urgency

Urgency is a desire to urinate that is sudden, forceful, and hard to ignore. When especially severe, this can be followed by *urgency incontinence,* or the involuntary loss of urine or leakage, preceded by a sudden urge to void that is so strong you "can't make it" to the bathroom. Urgency can be caused by disorders that make the bladder sensitive, such as a bladder infection or a bladder stone, or loss of the bladder's flexibility. The bladder's normally soft and accommodating muscular walls can become stiff and intolerant of filling when the nerves controlling urination are malfunctioning, or when it has overgrown its muscle bulk in an attempt to compensate for blockage. More will be said of this in chapter 5. In the absence of urinary tract problems, urgency and frequency can both be caused by anxiety.

Burning

The burning sensation that can accompany urination is usually due to inflammation or irritation of the delicate mucous membrane that lines the inside of the bladder and urethra. It is often associated with infection but can be due to other causes. Pain at the beginning of urination often results from inflammation in the urinary channel, or urethra, whereas pain at the end of urination is more likely to be caused by problems in the bladder. Irritation of the urethra where it passes through the prostate can also often cause a burning sensation, but the discomfort is usually felt at the tip of the penis.

Difficulty Starting Urination

Difficulty in starting the urinary stream can indicate blockage of the urethra due to prostate enlargement or narrowing of the urethra due to scar tissue. It can also occur when the bladder loses its ability to squeeze the urine out by muscular effort; this can be caused by diabetes, damage to the nerves controlling the bladder muscle, or damage to the bladder muscle itself from long-standing blockage. The same conditions can produce poor urinary stream flow as well as *intermittency*—spontaneous starting and stopping of the stream rather than uninterrupted flow. Some patients with blockage or loss of bladder strength complain of the need to strain or push to empty the bladder. This is often accompanied by a *feeling of incomplete emptying*—the sensation that urination has been incomplete. When the bladder fails to empty, *double voiding* can result. This is a need to urinate soon (ten to fifteen minutes) after voiding. *Dribbling at the end of urination* is an early symptom of prostate enlargement or blockage. It can be particularly bothersome to those who wear light-colored slacks.

Can Healthy Men Experience Difficulty Starting Urination?

Healthy men may have trouble starting to urinate in the presence of others. This is caused not by disease but by increased difficulty in pelvic floor relaxation due to nervousness and tension when there is a lack of privacy or strangers are present. Normally, it takes a few seconds to initiate the flow of urine—for the upper urethra to relax and change its shape from a closed tube to a funnel.

Repeated difficulty starting the urinary stream is one of the classic symptoms of prostate problems, so this complaint should be investigated, particularly when it occurs at home and in private. When benign overgrowth of the prostate results in alteration of the configuration or elasticity of the prostatic urethra, difficulty in beginning urination can result. Prostate cancer develops more peripherally in the prostate gland, not as close to the urethral channel. Consequently, prostate cancer may often be fairly advanced by the time it begins to cause difficulty with urination.

HOW CAN PROSTATE PROBLEMS CAUSE PAIN?

Pain can originate in the prostate itself, when infection causes swelling and inflammation. It is usually described as a dull, constant aching, located in the *perineum*—the region between the anal opening and the back of the scrotum. Pain originating in the prostate gland can radiate to (be felt in) the lower back, the groin, and even the legs. However, prostate swelling or enlargement due to tumors— either benign or malignant—usually does not cause pain.

Lower abdominal pain may occur when the prostate is infected or when a prostate infection leads to a bladder infection. The most common cause of lower abdominal pain in patients with prostate disorders is urinary retention: the bladder becomes painfully full, and urination is either impossible or too slow and trickling to effectively empty the bladder and relieve the pain. This backup of urine in the bladder due to blockage must occur fairly suddenly (over the course of days, not months) in order to cause pain. When weakness or neurologic paralysis of the bladder results in a similar backup that occurs over long periods of time, there is usually no pain.

When urinary retention occurs, the bladder enlarges enough to be felt as a firm rounded mass in the lower abdomen, just above the pubic bone. Every urologist has seen a patient who, while being evaluated for such a lower abdominal "tumor," is found to have a distended or blocked-up bladder. This condition is occasionally seen in a man with no symptoms of blockage and no abdominal pain. His only complaint is that he has had to switch from belts to suspenders. This case of *silent prostatism* is definitely the exception, however. Most men experience such uncomfortable symptoms while developing a blockage that they seek medical attention before the bladder has become damaged by severe and prolonged overstretching.

Back pain can have many urologic causes. When an infection in the urinary tract due to prostate blockage ascends into the kidney, pain high in the back on the affected side can occur. This is felt just below the lower ribs on one side or the other. Pain in the kidney can also be felt in the corresponding testicle because of the common origin of sensory nerves for both these structures. Testicular pain can also occur when infections in the bladder or prostate travel down the sperm ducts into the testicle and cause a painful condition called *epididymitis*. This is covered in more detail in chapter 4. As we

FIGURE 2-5
Back Pain Due to Prostate Cancer

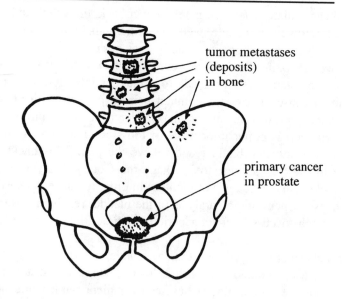

tumor metastases
(deposits)
in bone

primary cancer
in prostate

mentioned, pain in the prostate itself can be felt at times in the lower back. When prostate cancer in its later stages leaves the prostate and spreads into the body, it most commonly appears as secondary tumor deposits, or *metastases,* in the lower back bones. This causes severe continued back pain that can be disabling.

Blood in the urine should always be checked out, even though the majority of men who notice urinary bleeding don't have cancer. Nonetheless, this is the only warning given by malignant tumors of the urinary tract in some cases. When the entire urinary stream is bloody, the usual cause is bleeding from the kidneys, ureters, or bladder. Bleeding noticed only at the beginning or end of the urinary stream is more often due to a source in the prostate or urethra.

Blood in the semen usually results from minor inflammation of the prostate or seminal vesicles. It can be associated with prostate cancer, however, so it should be evaluated by a doctor. Fortunately, the majority of patients with this scary symptom will find that it goes away spontaneously and has no serious implications.

Urinary leakage, or *incontinence,* can be produced by a variety of conditions involving the prostate and lower urinary tract. *Urgency incontinence,* as described earlier in this section, is an urge to urinate so powerful and sudden that there is not enough time to get to the restroom before the loss of urine occurs. It can occur with infection or irritation of the bladder or prostate and in conditions that result in "residual urine," in which emptying of the bladder is incomplete.

Overflow incontinence occurs when the bladder stays nearly full all the time as a result of muscular weakness of the bladder wall, obstruction of the urethra, or both. The kidney adds steady output of urine into the bladder that can hold no more, and some "overflow" or leakage is pushed out of the urethra.

Total incontinence is steady leakage of urine that occurs all the time as a result of weakness or damage to the *sphincter,* the valve of the bladder. This form of incontinence is caused by serious neurologic malfunction, structural damage to the sphincter, surgery, or radiation.

Stress incontinence has nothing to do with mental stress. It occurs when the sphincter is weakened but still functional. This causes urinary leakage when the person coughs, sneezes, strains, lifts, laughs, or exercises. While stress incontinence can occur in some men following treatment for prostate cancer, it is much more common in women, in whom the cause is a gradual loss of support of the pelvic organs.

SEXUAL PROBLEMS

Male sexual dysfunction is often called *impotence,* although this term really refers to only the inability to get and keep an erection sufficiently hard or long-lasting for intercourse. As you can imagine, there is a wide range of severity. Some men get an erection that they cannot maintain, whereas others are unable to obtain an erection at all.

Loss of sexual desire can occur when blood levels of the male sex hormone, testosterone, are abnormally low. This low hormone level is deliberately created in men suffering advanced prostate cancer, because it slows tumor growth. If a patient experiences loss of desire, he should be checked to see if his hormone levels are normal. Loss of desire can also be a naturally adaptive mental response. When physical factors cause sexual problems, lessening of desire reduces frustration.

Absence of ejaculation during climax can have several causes. Following prostate surgery, anatomical changes in the upper urethra may allow semen discharged at climax to flow back into the bladder rather than forcefully exiting the penis in the usual manner (see figure 8–6). While this may change the sensation of ejaculation slightly, it is not harmful. Drugs for prostate enlargement may have this same effect. Surgery around the main blood vessels in the abdomen can also interfere with ejaculation, as can diabetes.

Premature ejaculation can be caused temporarily by irritation or inflammation in the lower urinary tract. When it occurs regularly, there may be psychological or emotional causes. When sex drive and erectile function are completely unimpaired, the *complete lack of orgasm* is usually related to psychological problems.

Chapter 3

═══════════

EXAMINATIONS AND TESTS

Lying as it does deep within the bones of the pelvis, the prostate is somewhat inaccessible. Its front side lies immediately behind the bridge of the "pubic bone" (actually the pubic symphysis) and therefore cannot be felt. The rectum wraps around the back of the prostate. If you have ever lain a sleeping bag over a large rock, you know that the size and shape of the rock can be felt in great detail. Similarly, the doctor's gloved finger can feel the prostate gland pushing itself against the front wall of the rectum.

The ability to feel the back, or posterior, part of the prostate through the wall of the rectum is the key to clinical examination of the prostate without using machinery. Our high-tech culture at times overlooks the simple tests, and this is one of the best. It is called the *digital rectal exam.* In electronics, "digital" (referring to sophisticated signal processing by numerical quantification) also originates from the Latin word for "finger"—in this sense the original unit for counting. I have to chuckle when one of my scientifically sophisticated patients, having read about a "digital" rectal exam, comes in expecting some type of electronic monitoring process.

The rectal exam is less than sophisticated, and therein lies the problem. It is somewhat crude and uncomfortable. Unlike women, who have to accustom themselves to pelvic examinations, men have had little or no experience with medical personnel poking into their bodily orifices. For this reason, most patients (especially younger

FIGURE 3-1
Rectal Exam

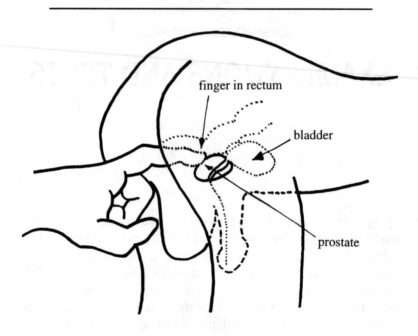

men) may find the rectal exam scary, embarrassing, degrading, humiliating, and uncomfortable. Unfortunately, these reactions prevent men from coming in for a prostate examination. While working at a free clinic set up to screen men for prostate cancer, I had one patient say, "Oh, you're not gonna do that, are you?" Unfortunately, he left once I told him that the examination wasn't mandatory. It is normal to complain about this test and express your distaste for it, but it remains the single most effective examination for detecting prostate cancer.

By sliding a gloved finger covered with sterile lubricant about an inch and a half into the rectum, the physician can feel most of the posterior, or rearward, "peripheral zone" of the prostate. This is the region where over 90 percent of prostate cancers originate. Although the anterior, or front, surface of the prostate can't be felt, it contains very little glandular tissue and therefore is not frequently involved in prostate cancer. Normally the prostate is about as big as a walnut and has the same rubbery consistency as the fleshy base of the thumb. In contrast, cancer within the prostate feels hard, more like the bony knuckle on the other side of the thumb. When prostate infection is present, mild pressure on the prostate during rectal exam may push a drop or two of prostate fluid into the urethra, where it can be collected at its opening. When this fluid is examined microscopically, signs of infection can often be detected.

EXAMINING THE REST OF THE URINARY TRACT

The abdominal exam allows a doctor to detect signs of bladder distention, or enlargement, that occurs when the bladder fails to empty normally. In addition, the uppermost part of the lower back, just below the lowest ribs on each side, is felt for any tenderness—a sign that urinary tract infection has involved the kidney or that blockage of the kidney has occurred.

Infection can also spread downward from the prostate into the testicles, so the physician usually checks here as well. The testes should be smooth oval structures with no major lumps or bumps. Occasionally the patient can feel a small nodular area where the sperm duct (or epididymis) is attached to the testicle, and this makes him worry about a tumor. This sperm duct is normally a soft structure running down the back of the testicle, but when it becomes infected it can become firm and very tender to touch.

Usually the groin areas are checked to detect weakness or bulging of the abdominal wall where it parts to let the cord through as it runs down to the testicle. This protrusion through the weak part of the abdominal wall, or *hernia*, can occur more often in men with severe symptoms of prostate blockage. By constantly straining and pushing to urinate, they increase their chances of developing a hernia. It is standard procedure to check a man with a hernia for prostate problems. If the hernia is repaired and the man continues to strain or push to urinate, there is a higher chance that the surgical repair will eventually fail.

HOW ARE LABORATORY TESTS USED TO CHECK
FOR PROSTATE DISEASE?

Laboratory tests are undertaken to answer questions raised by specific symptoms or to clarify findings discovered during an examination. The exceptions to this practice are tests used for screening the population at large; these laboratory tests themselves constitute valuable and reliable indicators of disease. More details about these tests will be given in chapter 6.

WHAT DOES URINALYSIS SHOW?

Routine testing of the urine involves two phases. First, a few chemical tests are performed by use of a *dipstick,* or paper strip of test patches. Observation of the color changes on the dipstick reveals the level of acidity in the urine, the presence of protein (an indicator of kidney disease), and the presence of sugar (a test for diabetes). Second, the urine is examined under a microscope for cells or bacteria.

The composition of urine under the microscope depends somewhat on how the urine is collected. The first bit of voided urine may contain whatever cellular debris or bacteria have contaminated the outer parts of the urethra. The urine flowing out at midstream is more representative of the urine in the kidneys and bladder. For this reason, examination of the first bit of urine voided is useful in detecting inflammation in the urethra or prostate.

Inflammation is the body's response to infection, trauma, or injury. It starts the healing process and is characterized by the accumulation of white blood cells in the inflamed area. When the urinary tract is infected, reaction to bacterial growth in the urine calls forth the ''shock troops'' of white blood cells in the membrane lining the urinary tract. These cells then appear in the urine. White blood cells can also be found in the urine in response to cancer or stones in the urinary tract, or as part of the healing process following surgery on the urinary tract. Normally, fewer than two white blood cells appear in the amount of urine displayed for microscope examination.

Red blood cells are often seen in the urinary tract in response to injury. They frequently are present in infection. Often they are the first finding that leads to the diagnosis of stones, cancer, or kidney disease. Normally, fewer than two red blood cells are seen per microscopic field.

Examination of the prostate fluid and semen is an important part of evaluating the patient with prostate infections or infertility. These problems are covered in greater detail in the following chapter.

BLOOD TESTS

The modern clinical laboratory can run hundreds of tests on a sample of blood. A few special tests are of particular importance to the evaluation of prostate disorders.

Kidney Function

Blockage of the urinary tract due to prostate enlargement can cause the kidneys to fail. Measurement of two substances in the blood normally excreted by the kidney along with its other waste products provides a measure of the kidney's filtration function.

Urea is produced by protein metabolism and is excreted by the kidneys. The *blood urea nitrogen (BUN)* test measures the quantity of urea in the blood. When the level of BUN rises abnormally high, it indicates that the kidneys are not doing their job to properly filter the blood. Variations in the BUN, however, can also occur because of dehydration, and therefore the test is not as accurate an indicator of kidney function as is the *serum creatinine*. Creatinine is a chemical compound produced by the body's muscles. Elevations of the creatinine level in blood specifically indicate reduction in the filtration function of the kidney. The overall performance of the kidney can be expressed as a number, the *creatinine clearance*, which represents the number of milliliters of blood that are completely cleared of creatinine each minute and is a good measure of filtration. The normal creatinine clearance is about 120 milliliters per minute. The body can survive on a wide range of creatinine clearance, but a certain minimum is necessary. Depending on dietary and fluid intake, *dialysis* (use of a "kidney machine" to filter the blood) is necessary to prevent death when the creatinine clearance drops lower than about 10 milliliters per minute.

Monitoring Tumors with Blood Tests

A great deal of research has been done to determine how a tumor grows, what is unique about a cancer cell, and how it differs from normal cells. Because all cancers are different, a single, simple measurable pattern, based on our current level of understanding, does not yet exist. It would be helpful if there were a single special protein or product found in the blood of anyone with cancer. While this would produce nightmare scenarios in those patients with a positive blood test but no detectable tumors, it would certainly aid in the early diagnosis of the disease.

Fortunately, there is a relatively new tool for diagnosing and monitoring prostate cancer. Based on the measurement of a protein produced only by the prostate, it is a blood test called the prostate-specific antigen, or PSA. A protein unique to semen was first identified in 1971, which was subsequently shown to be the product of only prostate cells. Later named gamma seminoprotein, it was studied by crime-lab researchers looking for a substance that could be used legally to prove the presence of semen. Antigen is the target substance in an antibody reaction, so when an accurate antibody test for gamma seminoprotein was developed, its concentration in the blood became known as the prostate-specific antigen level.

From its origins in crime detection, it is now being used to track another culprit: prostate cancer. In the diagnosis of prostate cancer, PSA is not perfectly accurate, as it also measures conditions other than cancer. Many patients with elevated PSA levels do not seem to have cancer. Five to ten percent of patients with prostate cancer may have a PSA level in the normal range. In patients known to have cancer, PSA provides an excellent index of their progress and response to therapy. Despite its shortcomings, PSA is the single most valuable blood test in the diagnosis and management of patients with prostate cancer today. The use of this test will be covered in greater detail in chapter 6.

IMAGES OF THE BODY

We take X-ray pictures for granted. The ability to study internal anatomy without using a knife has expanded so dramatically in recent years that the once miraculous X-rays have taken their place as just one of many different imaging techniques.

X-rays are a type of high-energy radiation similar to visible light but stronger. They are energetic enough to penetrate through many materials. The shadow cast by X-ray illumination yields various shades of gray, depending on how easily the rays penetrate a given type of tissue. In general, soft tissues allow X-rays to pass through, whereas bones don't. In order to allow visualization of soft tissue detail such as the configuration of the urinary tract, dyes, or *contrast agents,* are used. These substances do not permit free passage of the X-ray beam and therefore create bright shadows on the X-ray film similar to those created by bones.

X-ray energy does more than form pictures of living structures; it affects the structure itself. Although the dose received is minimal in most routine examinations, X-rays can be used to kill cells that make up tumors. X-rays remain a valuable diagnostic tool in many situations; when the situation demands, the benefits must be weighed against whatever risks are inherent in their use. Usually there are no significant risks from the minor exposures that accompany a normal X-ray examination.

The *intravenous pyelogram (IVP)* has been the standard X-ray examination of the urinary tract. In the last ten years, the number of IVPs done has decreased as other methods of looking at the urinary tract have evolved. It still remains the best initial examination of a patient suspected of having kidney or bladder stones. An IVP requires the intravenous administration of a contrast agent. This is usually an iodine-containing chemical that is filtered by the kidneys. When it is concentrated in the urinary tract by the kidneys, it causes the urinary tract to *opacify,* or appear white. This effectively outlines the urine-filled ducts of the kidney, the ureters, and the bladder, allowing the urinary tract to be easily seen on an X-ray.

FIGURE 3-2
IVP (Intravenous Pyelogram)

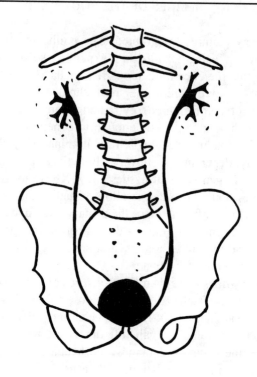

In the past, an IVP was routine in patients with prostate disorders. It allowed the doctor to assess how much blockage was present by measuring the residual urine present in the bladder after voiding. In addition, the degree of irregularity, or *trabeculation*, of the bladder could be assessed. Muscle thickening of the bladder due to obstruction causes this irregularity, and it can be seen during an IVP when the bladder fills with the X-ray dye. Normally, when the bladder is filled with dye, the interior lining gives off a relatively smooth, round shadow. In the presence of an obstruction, the shape of the bladder becomes irregular.

A *cystogram* is an X-ray made by instilling the X-ray dye directly into the bladder. It will not outline the kidneys or ureters, unless the ureters abnormally allow dye from the bladder to ascend up into the kidneys. This is called reflux and is not normal. Usually the ureters form a one-way valve where they enter the bladder—urine can go down into the bladder from the ureters, but when the bladder contracts during voiding, urine will not go up the ureter.

For examination of the bladder itself, the cystogram has an advantage over the IVP in that no intravenous dye injection need be given. With the use of intravenous X-ray dyes, there is a risk of allergic reaction to the dye as well as the possibility of dye-induced injury to the kidneys. This is particularly a problem in elderly patients and patients with advanced diabetes or other preexisting kidney diseases. These risks are avoided in the cystogram, wherein dye is instilled directly into the bladder through a catheter (a rubber tube inserted into the bladder through the opening of the penis). A cystogram is often obtained in a man who has required placement of a

FIGURE 3-3
Cystogram

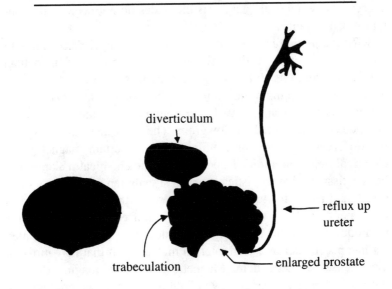

diverticulum

reflux up
ureter

trabeculation

enlarged prostate

normal bladder   obstructed bladder

catheter for the inability to urinate. In this patient, the cystogram provides information about prostate size, the degree of bladder irregularity or trabeculation suggestive of long-standing obstruction, and the presence of bladder stones that can form when the prostate obstructs urinary outflow.

Also, with the bladder full of dye, the catheter can be removed and a repeat X-ray taken after voiding. This permits the doctor to see how well the patient can void out the dye and empty the bladder.

CAT scan stands for *computerized axial tomography*. Tomography means taking X-rays of slices, or sections, of the body. It is an ingenious method that uses a combination of X-rays passed in various directions through sections of the body, and a complex mathematical calculation to "reconstruct" an image from the process. In prostate cancer, CAT scanning can be used to assess the size and extent of a prostate tumor.

Enlarged lymph nodes in certain areas may indicate that the cancer has spread, but this cannot be accurately determined by scans alone. CAT scans will not usually pick up lymph nodes smaller than 1 centimeter. Some of these very small lymph nodes can contain cancer, and, conversely, large visible nodes do not necessarily contain prostate cancer.

MRI (magnetic resonance imaging) is similar to CAT scanning in that it creates cross-sectional images, but it is more refined than CAT scanning in its ability to pick up changes in soft tissue appearance. CAT scanning relies only on the relative transparency of various tissues to an X-ray beam, and presents the results as a computer-reconstructed shadowgram. The MRI takes advantage of the different responses of atomic nuclei to certain magnetic and electrical field conditions. Depending on the chemical makeup of a body's tissues, characteristic electrical signals can be received, measured, and reconstructed into a picture when the tissue is placed in a magnetic field and then pulsed with radiofrequency energy. This technique appears to be quite safe, unless you have an implanted cardiac pacemaker or a vital internal metallic part that may move in the intense magnetic field. Magnetic resonance imaging uses no X-rays, utilizing a lower energy radiation similar to that produced by radio transmission. Unlike the uniform cross-sections created by

FIGURE 3-4
CAT Scan of Pelvis with Prostate Tumor

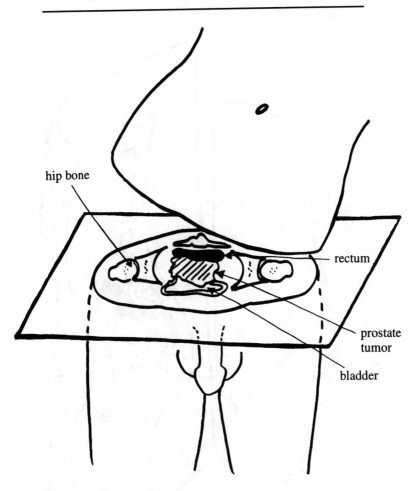

CAT scanning, magnetic resonance signals can be reconstructed into slices in any orientation: across the body, along the body's axis, or in an oblique direction.

Although MRIs and CAT scans compete to some degree for the same imaging tasks, magnetic resonance imaging is two to three times as costly as CAT scanning. MRI is accurate in evaluating the

FIGURE 3-5
MRI Scan

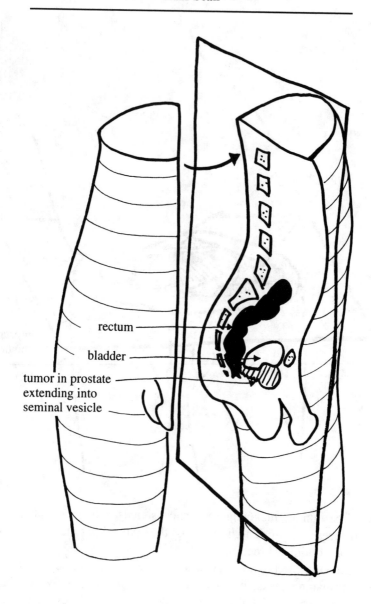

rectum

bladder

tumor in prostate
extending into
seminal vesicle

anatomic extent of prostate cancer, which provides help in clinically *staging* (establishing the anatomical extent of a tumor) this condition without surgery. MRI is of great benefit in evaluating problems of the back, arm, or leg in men with prostate cancer that has spread to the bones. Because it can "see" ligaments and soft tissues, rather than just bones, it is the examination of choice for knee and other joint injuries.

Bone scans are screening tests done in patients with prostate cancer to search for evidence of tumor spread. When cancer cells leave the prostate and spread through the body's lymphatic or vascular channels, they seem to prefer taking up residence in the bones. Medically, we say prostate cancer usually *metastasizes* to the bones. Bone scans are started by giving the patient an intravenous injection of a mix containing a minimal amount of a radioactive tracer. This is usually *technetium 99*, a compound that gradually undergoes transformation into an inert substance while creating a small amount of detectable radioactive energy. This compound is taken up by the body's bones, particularly in areas of bone that are inflamed, healing, or reacting to some stimulus. After the injection, a sensitive detector, called a gamma camera, is used to pick up the signals from this tracer and create an image. Any areas of bones harboring tumor will produce a "hot spot" on the scan. Arthritis, infections, or old areas of bone injury may also show up on the scan. It often takes the expertise of a radiologist to decide which lesions on a bone scan are significant.

Searching with Sound

Ultrasound imaging has shown dramatic growth in its application and technical quality in the last dozen years. It has grown to the point now where it has surpassed X-rays as the most common form of imaging used in the urologist's office today. In fact, ultrasound is probably the most common diagnostic imaging study of the urinary tract performed in any institution.

When Paul Langevin invented sonar (a method of detecting submerged obstacles by sending and receiving sound signals from on board ships) in 1917, he surely never imagined how useful this technique could be. The frequency of sound waves is related to their pitch, when they are in the audible range: Lower-frequency sounds have a lower pitch. *Ultrasound* refers to the higher frequencies of sound waves, which are inaudible. Different types of ultrasound energy have different characteristics. The lower ultrasound frequencies (around 4,000 cycles per second) penetrate well into tissue but produce fuzzy pictures when bounced back to the instrument by the body. Higher ultrasound frequencies (between 7,000 and 10,000 cycles per second) provide clearer pictures but penetrate less well into tissue. Depending on the clinical situation, the doctor must choose the most appropriate type of ultrasound.

Ultrasound can be delivered *transabdominally,* through the skin of the abdomen and flanks, or *transrectally,* directly into the prostate from a finger-shaped *transducer* placed in the rectum. Transrectal

FIGURE 3-6
Transrectal Ultrasound

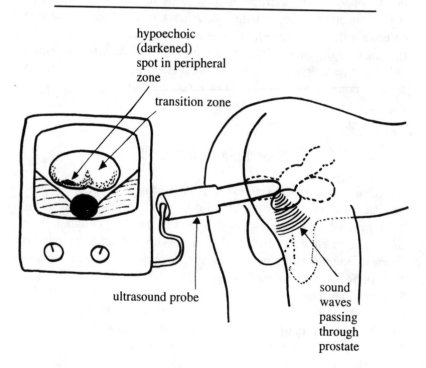

hypoechoic
(darkened)
spot in peripheral
zone

transition zone

ultrasound probe

sound
waves
passing
through
prostate

ultrasound is a preferred method for evaluating men for prostate cancer when other factors raise this suspicion. It is able to display the seminal vesicles and to distinguish the various anatomical zones of the prostate, including the peripheral zone, where cancers are most common. Prostate cancer usually produces a *hypoechoic* (dark) area in the peripheral zone.

Most transrectal ultrasound transducers have the capacity to accept a thin biopsy needle. By use of special software incorporated into the machine, the path that the needle takes through the tissue is shown on the display screen. When this path is directed through an abnormality seen on the screen, the needle can remove a small piece of tissue, or *biopsy* specimen, from this area for examination and analysis.

FIGURE 3-7
Ultrasound of Kidney

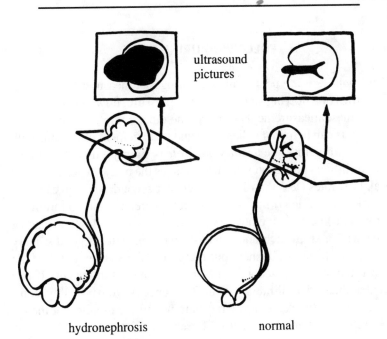

ultrasound pictures

hydronephrosis   normal

Transabdominal ultrasound is very helpful in evaluating how well the bladder empties. When an ultrasound examination of the bladder is performed immediately after urination (when the bladder should be fairly empty), the size of the bladder can easily be used to calculate the *residual urine*. This is fortunately replacing catheterization, or passage of a rubber tube into the bladder after urination, to measure residual urine. That technique was uncomfortable in the best case and could cause infection, bleeding, or urethral injury in the worst.

Ultrasound examination of the kidneys is a particularly safe and effective method for detecting changes in the upper urinary tract that can accompany prostate disorders. For example, severe prolonged blockage of the bladder due to prostate enlargement (benign or malignant) can produce backing up of the urine into the kidneys, or *hydronephrosis.*

In this condition the urinary ducts within the kidney balloon up, filling the kidney with urine that normally would freely drain down into the bladder.

FOLLOWING URINE FLOW

Urodynamics is a type of urologic testing that measures the physical properties of a flowing stream of urine: pressure, flow rate, and so on. While these measurements can become quite complex, simple measurements can help in the diagnosis and management of patients with prostate problems. The *urinary flow rate* is simply a measure of how fast (milliliters per second) the urine leaves the body. In general, slow peak flow rates (less than 12 milliliters per second) are suggestive of obstruction, while normal peak flow rates (greater than 15 milliliters per second) help to rule out this problem. A simple flow rate can be done with a stopwatch and a measuring cup. After a good urinary stream has been established, put the cup in the stream and start the stopwatch. After six seconds, measure the amount in the cup. If it is greater than 75 milliliters (about 2.5 ounces), you probably don't have a major blockage. Flow rates are useful for monitoring the response of prostate blockage to different medications.

LOOKING INSIDE—ENDOSCOPY

Today, many surgeons use sophisticated scopes and optical systems
to perform surgery without making an incision. Urologic surgeons
were pioneers in this regard, dating back to the invention of the
cystoscope (bladder-scope).

There are a variety of ways to look in the urinary tract. Fortu-

FIGURE 3-8
Cystoscope

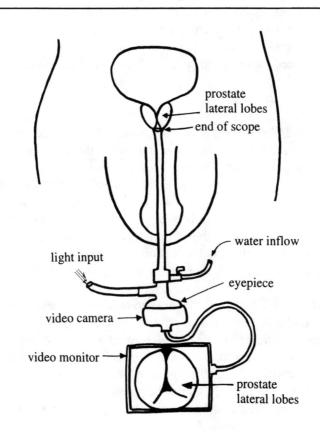

nately, several noninvasive alternative tests make cystoscopy less common than it was in the past. With the increasing use of ultrasound bladder residuals and flow rates, there is less need to look at the prostate in order to diagnose obstruction. Cystoscopy remains an important test in evaluating the cause of blood in the urine, and it is employed (when the patient is under anesthesia) in some methods of prostate surgery.

SENDING A LITTLE PIECE OF YOU TO THE LAB

Prostate biopsy is necessary for the definitive diagnosis of prostate cancer. It can be done in either of three ways: *transrectal, transperineal,* or *transurethral.* When a transrectal biopsy is done as part of a transrectal ultrasound examination, the thin biopsy needle punctures the rectal wall in the process. This part of the rectal wall has no nerve fibers to sense this type of sharp pain, so the sensation is bothersome but usually not painful. An automatic device enables the needle to shave out a tiny sliver of prostate tissue, all in a fraction of a second. As in the case of any biopsy, bleeding can be a risk. Since the needle penetrates the rectal wall, infection is also a risk, and antibiotics are usually given as a precaution.

Transperineal biopsy of the prostate usually involves a similar needle, but it passes into the prostate directly through the soft tissues of the *perineum,* the region between the scrotum and rectum. Since the needle does not enter the rectum, infection is much less likely in this technique. Digital guidance (doing the biopsy while a finger is feeling the nodule in the prostate) works well with the perineal approach.

Transurethral biopsy of the prostate is used in special situations: a patient who is suspected of having prostate cancer but who has undergone surgical removal of the rectum for colon cancer or other causes. When the prostate can't be felt, passage of a special scope while the patient is anesthetized can allow prostate tissue to be removed from the inside. This can be problematic, as is evident from our earlier anatomical discussions. The regions immediately surrounding the urethra are not generally at risk for prostate cancer, so these biopsies need to be rather extensive. More will be said of this technique in chapter 5, as it is more commonly utilized as a method for removing benign prostate overgrowth in men with urinary blockage.

Chapter 4

PROSTATE PROBLEMS IN THE YOUNGER MAN— Prostatitis and Infertility

Frederick B. is a forty-five-year-old commodities broker, healthy and active in sports. Recently, he had been seen by his family doctor, who referred him to me when his condition wouldn't clear up.

"It started last summer, Doctor. I came home from Montana, and I noticed that I'm getting up two or three times every night to urinate. I never used to. The urine flow seems slower as well. I've been on three different antibiotics, and none of them seem to help."

Rather than asking about blood in the urine, or burning, I asked him about the trip. It turned out that he had been cycling through the Flathead Valley, and we ended up discussing the differences between mountain and road bikes. Finally, Frederick told me what was bothering him.

"I've been told I have prostatitis, and it just isn't getting any better. I'm worried it may be causing some real damage."

Frederick's examination showed that his prostate was tender, which could have been caused by his long bike ride. However, a drop of prostate fluid that came out of the urinary channel after the examination showed small amounts of white blood cells. I reviewed his previous records; cultures of his urine and prostate fluid had grown no bacteria or other microorganisms. There was no infection at this time, and I related this to him.

"I don't get it, Doctor—if there's no infection, why have I been taking antibiotics? Isn't prostatitis infection of the prostate gland?"

The intensive care unit nurse called me, because she had not previously admitted a patient to the unit with a diagnosis of acute bacterial prostatitis. Unlike Frederick B., Anthony had positive urine cultures. In addition, incubation of his blood in a special nutrient broth produced the same bacterial organisms that were present in the urine.

"I'm turning down his intravenous rate until you can get over here," the nurse told me on the phone. "His bladder seems to be getting distended."

Enough swelling had taken place in Anthony's prostate to compress the urinary channel and make it impossible for him to urinate. We had been giving him IV fluids at a good clip, as his blood pressure was a little low and he needed the extra volume in his blood vessels. Sometimes, bacterial infection in the blood stream can cause the blood pressure to drop, and the patient will go into *septic shock.* If this is allowed to persist, low blood pressure levels can cause kidney damage. Fortunately, Anthony's kidneys were working well. They had filled the bladder with more urine than it could flush out through his blocked urethra.

I had to go into the hospital and place a *suprapubic tube* (see Figure 4–3). This catheter, with the aid of a little local anesthetic, is inserted into the bladder directly through the skin of the lower abdomen to avoid passing through the urinary channel. Placing one in the usual manner—sliding it up the urethra—would have been out of the question. His prostate was so tender that a urethral catheter would have caused him constant pain.

WHAT IS PROSTATITIS?

Prostatitis is inflammation of the prostate gland, and it is a very broad and inclusive term. Patients with prostatitis range from men with vague discomfort and urinary symptoms originating in this region, without clear-cut laboratory evidence of disease, to individuals with a virulent bacterial infection.

WHAT ARE THE SYMPTOMS OF PROSTATITIS?

Prostatitis usually causes discomfort in and around the prostate, and urinary complaints. In severe cases, usually involving a dangerous degree of bacterial infection, more *systemic,* or "whole body," symptoms may appear. These can include fever, chills, muscle or joint aching, back pain, nausea, or disorientation.

Pain from prostatitis can be perceived as perineal pain (between the rectum and back side of the scrotum), low back pain, suprapubic pain (just above the pubic bone), lower abdominal pain, groin pain, or pain in the testicles. Occasionally pain is felt at the tip of the penis, but usually this is present only during urination.

The effects of prostate inflammation on urinary tract function include frequent urination, the urgent desire to void, and increased

FIGURE 4-1
Compression of Urethra

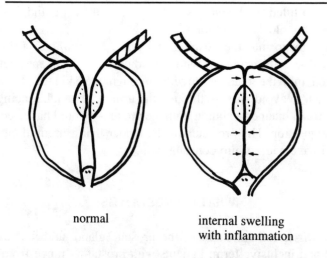

normal

internal swelling
with inflammation

nighttime voiding. The desire to void may be felt and rapidly becomes painfully urgent, only to fade away when the patient gets to the restroom and is unable to void. Because of an unyielding "capsule" around the gland, inflammation and swelling within the prostate may cause compression of the urethra and obstruction of urinary flow. Patients often complain of slowing of the stream, hesitancy, or a "stop-and-start" stream. Occasionally they have a sensation of incomplete emptying.

Inflammation

Inflammation is a response to infection or injury, which choreographs the blood vessel changes and cellular activity necessary to protect the body and permit healing. It initiates a carefully regulated series of defense strategies that destroy invading microorganisms, then sets the stage for healing and repair of injured tissue.

Although inflammation is created and regulated by subtle chemical messages and control signals, its overall effects have been detectable by physicians for hundreds of years. Heat, redness, swelling, and pain are the classic hallmarks of inflammation. Heat and redness occur when the blood vessels dilate, or open up, while swelling results from blood vessels becoming less "watertight" and leaking fluid out into the surrounding tissues. Pain occurs in response to pressure on nerve endings from swelling and is also the direct effect of some of the chemical messengers involved in inflammation on the nerve endings.

In prostatitis, inflammation of the prostate gland produces swelling (which secondarily chokes off the urinary channel) and pain. The increased "leakiness," or permeability, of the blood vessels in the area, and the attraction of white blood cells to an area of inflammation, result in the entrance of white blood cells into the urethra and glandular chambers of the prostate. Fluid coming from the prostate, such as the first few drops of urine voided, or the fluid expressed from the prostate during examination, will contain white blood cells when inflammation is present.

FIGURE 4-2
Effects of Inflammation

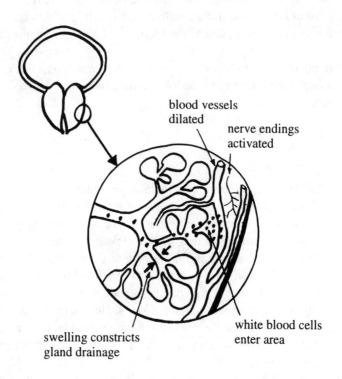

blood vessels
dilated

nerve endings
activated

swelling constricts
gland drainage

white blood cells
enter area

Infection

The inflammation characteristic of prostatitis can be brought on in some cases by infection of the prostate gland with bacteria or other microorganisms. What is infection? It occurs when bacteria or other disease-causing creatures take over bodily tissues by growing where they shouldn't. Bacteria are present on everyone's skin, but it would be incorrect to say that everyone is "infected." Infection implies an abnormal overgrowth accompanied by some reaction or symptoms in its victim. Because of this distinction, we usually try to determine how many bacteria are present. In the case of urine, for instance, most doctors look for more than one hundred thousand bacteria per milliliter of urine to prove infection is present. As we will see, this numerical criterion may not always be appropriate in patients with prostatitis.

When urine is obtained, it is "plated," or spread upon a plate containing a layer of agar, a special nutrient gel that allows bacteria to grow. The plate is then placed in an incubator and inspected after twenty-four hours to determine whether any growth has occurred. When bacteria are present in the urine, each cell landing on the agar will multiply into a small colony of bacteria that will be visible to the naked eye twenty-four hours later. By taking into account the volume of urine that has been plated, it is possible to determine how many colonies are present per milliliter of urine.

HOW IS URINE COLLECTED IN MEN WITH SUSPECTED INFECTION, AND WHAT DOES IT TELL US?

Whoever has been told to "pee in a jar" at the doctor's office knows there is no big trick to this. When prostate infection is suspected, however, the method of collection is different. It is known that in men with bacterial infection of the prostate, urine voided immediately after a digital rectal exam will contain the causative bacteria. A systematic method for pinpointing the source of urinary infections in men involves separate collection of different parts of the stream. The initial voided specimen is collected in one cup and termed *VB-1,* the midstream specimen is collected separately and termed *VB-2,* and the urine collected after digital rectal exam is termed *VB-3.* Appropriately, this process is termed a *three-glass urinalysis.*

In the presence of a bladder infection, the bacterial counts in VB-2 and VB-3 will be about the same. In true bacterial infection of the prostate gland, VB-3 will have a higher count than VB-2. Moreover, to establish a diagnosis of bacterial prostatitis, the VB-3 counts must exceed the urethral or VB-1 counts by at least a factor of ten.

THE VARIETIES OF PROSTATITIS

When a man has symptoms originating in the prostate gland and laboratory evidence of inflammation, he will be diagnosed as having prostatitis. If bacteria can be cultured from the urine or prostate fluid, he has *bacterial prostatitis*. If inflammation is present but cultures grow no bacteria, the condition is called *abacterial* or *nonbacterial prostatitis*. If the symptoms alone are present, and there is no laboratory evidence of inflammation, the condition is more appropriately termed *prostatodynia*, which means pain in the prostate. In one study of over five hundred men with similar symptoms, 5 percent of men had bacterial prostatitis, 64 percent had nonbacterial prostatitis, and 31 percent were found to have prostatodynia.

THE MAGNITUDE OF THE PROBLEM

Men with symptoms due to an infected, inflamed, or unexplainably bothersome prostate are not uncommon in urologists' offices. The exact incidences of these various conditions are not known. Data from the National Center for Health Statistics show that in a given year there are approximately twenty annual office visits per one thousand men for prostatitis. The syndrome is most common in younger men; a man under fifty who is seeking medical care for problems involving his prostate most likely has some variation of prostatitis or prostatodynia.

ACUTE BACTERIAL PROSTATITIS

This is the most clear-cut example of prostate infection, and is definitely the most dangerous. Fortunately, it is also the least common form of prostatitis—most clinics see less than 5 percent of prostatitis patients with this diagnosis.

Typically, the patient rapidly is taken ill, with malaise (feeling poorly) and back and perineal pain associated with fever and shaking chills. Urination is usually slowed, and patients note increased frequency, urgency, and burning or pain with urination.

A rectal examination of the prostate must be done very gently and carefully in this situation. Undue squeezing or compression of the prostate to obtain specimens may result in spreading infection to the bloodstream. The prostate is usually very tender, making the rectal exam very uncomfortable. Even without a rectal exam, some patients with acute bacterial prostatitis have positive blood cultures for bacteria, showing that the infection has spread out of the prostate and into the bloodstream. The urine within the bladder usually becomes infected, which makes identification of the exact bacteria type present fairly straightforward by a simple urine culture. This information is critically important in the patient with an aggressive bacterial infection, as it serves to identify what type of antibiotic will be effective in promptly clearing the condition.

Patients with acute bacterial prostatitis frequently require hospitalization for administration of intravenous antibiotics. When oral antibiotic therapy is appropriate, the most commonly used drugs are trimethoprim-sulfa, carbenicillin, ciprofloxacin, lomefloxacin, and orofloxacin.

When acute bacterial prostatitis results in severe restriction of urine flow due to prostatic swelling, a special type of catheter is generally used—the *percutaneous suprapubic tube.* Percutaneous means placed directly through the skin, while suprapubic refers to the fact that it enters the bladder above the pubic bone. With an acutely inflamed and infected prostate surrounding the upper part of the urethra, a standard catheter passing through the urethra is intolerably uncomfortable.

Surprisingly, a small caliber suprapubic catheter generally causes very little discomfort.

Most patients with acute bacterial prostatitis can be given oral antibiotics a day or two after their temperature comes down to normal as they receive intravenous antibiotics. If the temperature remains normal for twenty-four hours after the start of oral antibiotics, the patient can be discharged from the hospital.

Usually, there are no long-lasting aftereffects or complications from acute bacterial prostatitis. However, in some cases the bacteria may not be completely eradicated, which can lead to chronic or recurring bacterial prostatitis.

Occasionally, acute bacterial prostatitis can lead to a *prostatic abscess,* wherein the inflammation associated with infection results in destruction of some of the body's own tissues. This creates a walled-off cavity containing sloughed or dead tissues and bacteria, which usually requires surgical drainage.

FIGURE 4-3
Catheters

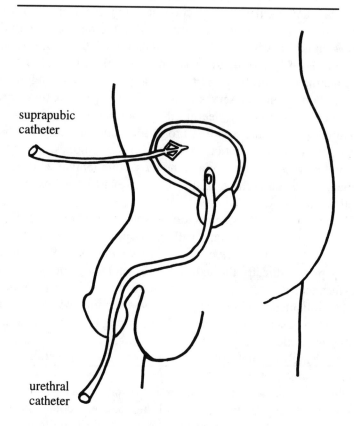

suprapubic
catheter

urethral
catheter

CHRONIC BACTERIAL PROSTATITIS

This bacterial infection of the prostate is less severe than acute
bacterial prostatitis. It is often the cause of recurring urinary infections in men, when infection of prostate fluids spreads to the urine
inside the bladder.

FIGURE 4-4
Abscess in Prostate

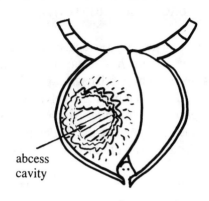

abcess
cavity

CAN MEN HAVE INFECTED URINE AND NOT KNOW IT?

Yes, although nonsymptomatic urinary infection in men is uncommon. In one study of over a thousand men without pain or burning, no patients were found to harbor infection when they were younger than forty-nine years of age. In men between fifty and sixty, 0.6 percent were infected, while in men between sixty and seventy, 1.5 percent were infected. In men over age seventy, 3.6 percent were found to harbor urinary infection but had no symptoms.

Chronic bacterial prostatitis may be the source of nonsymptomatic bacterial urinary infection, but most men with chronic bacterial prostatitis have symptoms. They are low abdominal or perineal pain; pain that radiates into the groin, testes, or penis; or pain that occurs after ejaculation. Symptoms of bladder irritation (such as frequency, urgency, or burning with urination) are usually present. Prostate inflammation can cause slowing of the urinary stream, although complete blockage is much less common than in acute bacterial prostatitis. Occasionally, bloody semen is caused by chronic bacterial prostatitis.

WHAT TESTS ARE REQUIRED TO DIAGNOSE CHRONIC BACTERIAL PROSTATITIS?

When the three-glass method proves bacterial infection is present in the prostate, and the patient has recurring episodes of pain and burning, the diagnosis of chronic bacterial prostatitis can be made. When medication fails, an X-ray of the pelvis and a prostate ultrasound may be helpful in determining whether stones are present in the prostate. With the passage of years, hardening of the minerals in prostate secretions or urine can produce small stones within prostate gland chambers or ducts.

These small stones can be found in most men who are middle-aged or older, and they usually are of no consequence, producing no symptoms or infection. If they happen to be present in an individual with chronic infection of the prostate, they can impair efforts to overcome infection with medication alone. Severe chronic bacterial prostatitis with prostate stones may be one of the few cases in which surgery is used to treat prostatitis.

FIGURE 4-5
Prostatitis with Stones

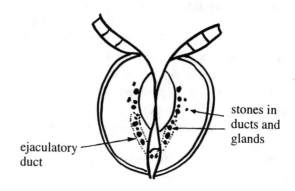

ejaculatory duct

stones in ducts and glands

DO MEN WITH CHRONIC PROSTATITIS HAVE ABNORMAL SEMEN?

There are certain patterns of chemical alteration in the prostate fluid of men with chronic bacterial prostatitis, although it is not known whether these alterations make a person more susceptible to infection, or are the secondary consequences of infection.

Prostatic fluid is normally mildly acidic. Most researchers agree that prostate fluid becomes less acidic with age, and the prostate fluid of men with chronic infection is less acidic than normal. Again, it is not known whether this is the cause or effect of infection.

In healthy men, a potent antibacterial substance is present in prostatic fluid that can easily kill most bacteria. However, it appears to be severely lacking or missing altogether in men with chronic bacterial infections. Zinc dissolved in the prostate fluid has been shown to be this antibacterial factor, which raises the question of nutritional therapy for chronic infection. However, studies have shown that oral zinc treatment does not seem to alter the abnormal zinc levels in these patients.

TREATMENT OF CHRONIC BACTERIAL PROSTATITIS

For an antibiotic pill to eliminate an infection, it must first be absorbed through the digestive tract, enter the bloodstream, and then be presented to the infected tissues or body fluids in high enough concentrations to kill bacteria. Research has shown that most antibiotics produce effective bacteria-killing levels in prostate tissues but that some antibiotics give greater concentration in prostate fluid than others. For this reason, not all oral antibiotics are prescribed to treat chronic bacterial prostatitis.

The antibiotics usually recommended are trimethoprim-sulfa, cephalexin, ciprofloxacin, norfloxacin, orofloxacin, lomefloxacin, erythromycin, minocycline, and doxycycline. Even with long-term therapy (four to sixteen weeks), cure rates of only 30 to 40 percent are reported. This means that 60 to 70 percent of patients with this condition will suffer relapses. If the relapses are few and far between, repeated treatment courses may be appropriate. For those patients who continue to have bacteria in the urine and persistent symptoms, it may be necessary to maintain control with daily small suppressive doses of medication. Trimethoprim-sulfa or nitrofurantoin is typically prescribed for this, as they do not foster the development of new, resistant bacteria.

Surgery is not usually warranted in the treatment of chronic bacterial prostatitis. It has been shown that transurethral resection of the prostate (see chapter 7 for the details of this procedure) will cure only about 30 percent of men with this condition. When prostate stones are present in someone with severe, debilitating chronic bacterial prostatitis, a very complete resection of all prostatic tissue by this technique in an effort to remove the infected stones may be helpful. Complete removal of the prostate, as is done for prostate cancer, is not warranted.

NONBACTERIAL PROSTATITIS

Although nonbacterial prostatitis is the most common variety of prostatitis, little is known about its cause. The hundreds of patients with this diagnosis that are seen every year in a busy urology clinic may find that their symptoms come and go with little regard for the treatments and medications prescribed by their doctors.

The symptoms of this condition are much the same as described in the previous section. In some cases, urinary symptoms are less, and pelvic or postejaculatory pain more prominent. Although the prostate may be tender on physical examination, and microscopic examination of prostate fluid reveals white blood cells, cultures of urine and prostate fluid are negative for bacteria. Studies on men with this disorder have failed to show any convincing pattern of infection with other microorganisms, such as *Chlamydia*. This is a specialized organism that requires growth within cells and is responsible for urethral and genital duct infection in men.

TREATMENT OF NONBACTERIAL PROSTATITIS

Treatment of nonbacterial prostatitis can be frustrating for both doctor and patient. Since there is no reliable indication that this problem is due to infection, repeated courses of different antibiotic medications are probably not warranted. When bacterial cultures prove negative, it may be reasonable to try a limited course of antibiotics directed at nonbacterial agents, such as *Chlamydia,* in the event that infection is present. Tetracycline, doxycycline, minocycline, erythromycin, or ciprofloxacin is usually prescribed. Again, when all patients with this diagnosis are taken as a group, there is no convincing evidence that *Chlamydia* infection is the cause.

The inflammation in nonbacterial prostatitis, revealed by the presence of white blood cells in the prostate fluid, is of unknown cause. Drugs active against inflammation may be helpful in alleviating some of the symptoms of this condition. Ibuprofen is often used, given at 600 to 800 milligrams three to four times per day. Hot baths are helpful in reducing inflammation, and normal sexual activity is not discouraged. Some patients improve when citrus products, spicy foods, and alcohol are restricted for a while, although this varies considerably from individual to individual.

When the symptoms of a disorder rather than an identified cause become the focus of treatment, frustration is bound to arise in both the patient and the doctor. Because of this, good communication and an unhurried, in-depth talk with your doctor regarding the nature of the condition are essential.

PAINFUL PROSTATE—PROSTATODYNIA

This bothersome condition has many of the symptoms of prostatitis but no evidence of infection or inflammation. The chief complaint is usually of pain coming from somewhere in the pelvic or genital region. As with other problems involving the prostate, urinary complaints are often present as well. Examination usually reveals little more than tenderness of the prostate and surrounding structures.

DO PATIENTS WITH THIS CONDITION HAVE
ANY MEASURABLE ABNORMALITY?

Research studies involving careful measurements and X-rays of the voiding process have shown abnormalities in patients with prostatodynia, including flow restriction due to increased muscle tension in the prostatic portion of the urethra. Alteration in flow and secondary increases in urinary pressure may allow urine to enter the ducts of the prostate gland and chemically incite symptoms. These complex tests are for research only; helping patients with prostatodynia does not usually require these expensive and invasive studies.

WHAT DO TENSION HEADACHES
AND PROSTATODYNIA HAVE IN COMMON?

Many patients with prostatodynia appear to have too much tension in the pelvic floor muscles. These muscles, which surround the prostate and rectum, are involved in the urinary and rectal sphincter, or closure, systems.

Excessive muscle tension can result in aching or discomfort in this region, just as periods of elevated muscle tension in the neck and scalp muscles can produce headaches. Psychological studies have shown that patients with prostatodynia are more likely to have bodily expression of anxiety and increased muscle tension. Physical factors can cause pain in the pelvis as well. Occasionally, cyclists spending many hours a week on a narrow racing seat may develop some of the symptoms of prostatodynia. Their problems are less likely to cause troublesome alterations in muscle tension, as their physical conditioning is much better than the average person.

TREATMENT OF PROSTATODYNIA

Studies have shown that treatments aimed at reducing the closure or spasm of the prostatic urethra may help patients with this problem.

FIGURE 4-6
Muscles Around the Prostate

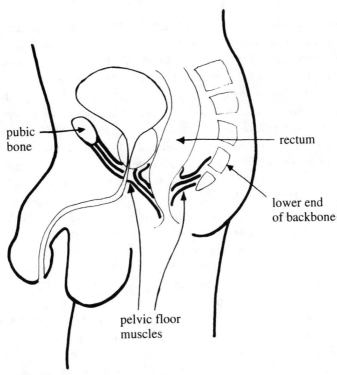

pubic
bone

rectum

lower end
of backbone

pelvic floor
muscles

There is a whole class of drugs called *alpha blockers* that reduce the
tension in the bladder neck and prostatic urethral muscles. One
medication, prazosin, helps to open the prostate and improve urinary
flow when given at about 2 milligrams per day. In some patients
with particularly debilitating symptoms who have not responded to
medication, physical stretching of the prostatic urethra and bladder
neck has been helpful. This procedure, called balloon dilation of the
prostate, involves inflation of a special balloon within the prostatic
urethra during anesthesia. Alpha blockers and balloon dilation are
described in greater detail in chapters 5 and 7.

Hot baths will help reduce discomfort during a flare-up. In patients with symptoms related to muscle tension, the limited use of
muscle relaxants such as diazepam may be helpful.

IS THE DOCTOR AWARE OF ALL MY CONCERNS?

A patient's anxiety seems to be related to the amount of uncertainty surrounding his diagnosis. When the clinical story includes an identifiable villain, such as disease-causing bacteria, everyone is comfortable as long as the proper therapy has been started. In conditions where the cause of symptoms is more complex or obscure, patients often remain anxious, and doctors may limit discussions so they do not have to emphasize the uncertainty of the cause. In many cases of nonbacterial prostatitis or prostatodynia, this lack of discussion may prevent the doctor from properly allaying the patient's concerns and anxieties. Reassurance that a condition is noninfectious, is not contagious, and does not lead to cancer or other serious complication is helpful but not enough. It is important that the doctor and patient review all the patient's concerns and carefully discuss whatever symptoms are present. This will not make the condition go away, but it usually will reduce the amount of discomfort and curtail much of the worry caused by a flare-up.

It is important to emphasize that prostate inflammation in the absence of infection (nonbacterial prostatitis), and prostate symptoms in the absence of inflammation (prostatodynia), are *not* "in your head." These are not imagined problems but real symptoms— often of unknown cause. Heightened awareness of sensations within the genital tract may be amplified by worry. In a person free of anxiety, the minor sensations that are probably felt at one time or another by most men can remain just that—minor sensations. When visits to a busy clinic result in a cursory discussion and repeated treatment with antibiotics, there is the possibility that something is being overlooked.

INFERTILITY

Infertility is another problem in younger men that can make the frustrations of recurrent prostatitis seem mild by comparison. About 15 percent of couples are unable to conceive within a one-year period of unprotected intercourse. In 20 percent of these couples, the male alone is at fault, whereas in 30 percent there are causes contributed by both partners. Therefore, about 50 percent of all infertile couples involve a male-related problem. Male infertility is a complicated subject, whose details are far beyond the scope of this book. However, a small segment of men may have fertility problems related to the prostate gland.

PROSTATE INFECTION AND INFERTILITY

The basic study in infertility is a semen analysis. Sperm counts normally should show greater than fifty million sperm per milliliter; a volume of semen of 1.5 to 5.0 milliliters; and motility, or motion, that appears to be present in greater than half of the sperm examined.

TABLE 4-1
Normal Semen

Volume	Sperm Count	Activity and Movement	Form
1.5–5 milliliters (⅓–1 tablespoon)	more than 50 million per milliliter	more than 60% of sperm cells are moving, with 10%–20% showing definite progression	more than 60% of sperm cells have normal shape or appearance

Studies by the World Health Organization have shown increased infertility or semen abnormalities in relation to genital tract infection in men. Despite this finding, no research has yet demonstrated a precise correlation between a given infection and reduced fertility. That means we do not know exactly how, or by what means, infection of the genital tract produces male infertility.

Patients who are being evaluated for infertility should be tested for genital tract infection if they show clinical evidence of inflammation in the urinary tract—, that is, any of the symptoms or laboratory findings of prostatitis described earlier, or the appearance of white blood cells in the semen specimen. Two specialized micro-organisms that are found in the genital tract, *Mycoplasma* and *Chlamydia*, don't always show themselves in routine bacterial cultures. Specialized tests for these infectious agents should also be done. When they are present, treatment involves antibiotic therapy with erythromycin, minocycline, doxycycline, or tetracycline.

GENITAL TRACT OBSTRUCTION WITHIN THE PROSTATE

About 10 percent of patients seen in infertility clinics don't merely have a low sperm count; they have *no* sperm present at all. This condition, *azoospermia,* can be due to one of two causes: either the testicle completely fails to produce sperm cells, or the duct system responsible for their transport into the urethra is not open. Some of these patients may have azoospermia due to obstruction of the ejaculatory ducts within the prostate.

FIGURE 4-7
Blockage of Ejaculatory Duct

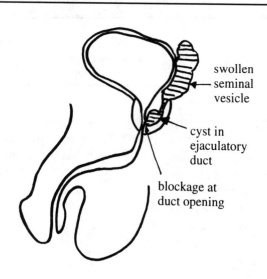

swollen
seminal
vesicle

cyst in
ejaculatory
duct

blockage at
duct opening

To recall the description in chapter 1, the ejaculatory ducts are the opening of the sperm transport system within the prostatic urethra. Evidence of their obstruction can be found with transrectal ultrasound. When a cyst in the area of the ejaculatory ducts is present, or the seminal vesicles are abnormally dilated in a patient with azoospermia and low semen volume, the diagnosis can be made. Treatment consists of removing a small amount of tissue where the ducts enter the urethra, using the resectoscopes (described in the following chapters) designed for prostate surgery. The rate of success with this type of surgery is very promising. In a recent study of twenty-four such patients, seven pregnancies were achieved after treatment.

EJACULATORY PROBLEMS

Ejaculatory difficulties rarely cause infertility. They can result from prostate surgery, although most men who need prostate surgery are past the age of interest in fertility. Ejaculation is a muscular phenomenon that coordinates contraction of the seminal vesicles and the ampullary ends of the vas deferens, and closure of the bladder neck. Various illnesses and injuries can prevent the bladder neck from closing. This allows the ejaculated semen to travel backward into the bladder (retrograde ejaculation) rather than out of the penis.

When retrograde ejaculation is the result of medical diseases such as diabetes mellitus or multiple sclerosis, drugs that bring about bladder neck closure can be used. When this problem is due to injuries or to surgical alteration of anatomy, it may be necessary to catheterize the patient after ejaculation and recover the semen from the bladder. After special treatment, the semen can then be used for artificial insemination.

Chapter 5

AGING AND THE PROSTATE—

Benign Prostatic Hypertrophy (BPH)

George A. finally came in to see me on his own, after his family doctor had been trying to set up an appointment with a urologist for the last two years. Getting up five or six times every night to go to the bathroom didn't really bother him, but one particular occurrence finally made him realize that something might be wrong.

"I've been waiting for my daughter to let me take my grandson to a baseball game. He's her first child and she is a little nervous about what he does. Well, she finally gave in.

"He's a pretty sturdy six-year-old, but with her worries on my mind, I just couldn't leave him sitting alone in the stands. The kid ended up spending more time in the men's room than watching the game.

"I didn't drink much at all, doc. Ten minutes after I left the john,

I felt like I had to go back. I was glad for the TV screens they have in the rest room, to keep up on the game when there's a crowd. But when I dropped Billy off at home, his mom wanted to know how he liked the ballpark. The little troublemaker said, 'Grandpa made me watch most of the game on the TV set in the bathroom.' "

Robert G. was like many of my other patients. He was fortunate to have been in fairly good health for his 83 years and came in at the insistence of his wife.

"She wants me to be checked because I got a dinky little spot on her car seat. We were already off the freeway, looking for a service station—but I couldn't quite hold it. It's happened a few times before, if I drank too much."

After I had examined him, we sat down to talk. I started explaining bladder obstruction to him and outlined the tests we might consider to see whether his blockage was serious enough to warrant treatment. I must have gotten carried away with my description of treatments and their side effects.

"Hold on, doctor. If you can convince my wife that I don't have cancer and I might live a little longer, we can forget this whole thing. It's not a bother, really. In fact, it will help me talk her into a motor home . . . with a bathroom."

Ernest came over to my house to pick up my fiddle for repair. He insisted, although I told him that it wasn't worth much, I could hardly play it, and I didn't think there was anything wrong with it.

"It is my great pleasure to do this for you," he said with a slight Austrian accent. Although he had retired years earlier, he was a skilled violin repairman. According to his wife, his ability to improve the sound of an instrument with a few minor adjustments was legendary. I listened as he went through a long list of obscure European violinists who had entrusted him with their instruments.

"Doctor, I am not unfamiliar with medical history. I can now understand why someone might submit to the pain and danger of bladder stone removal in the days before anesthesia and the germ theory of infection."

He had suffered from a near-medieval affliction with pain, burning, and uncontrollable spasms of the bladder. When microscopic blood was found in his urine, X-rays were taken and a bladder stone was found. This mineral deposit had resulted from the stagnation of urine in his bladder, caused by obstruction within the prostate. In addition to removal of the bladder stone, his surgery included prostate removal through a urethral endoscope.

Ernest was grateful after surgery. The best results often are obtained in patients with the most severe symptoms—someone who has forgotten what it is like to feel normal.

OVERVIEW

By the time a man reaches fifty he is likely to notice slowing of urinary flow. This extremely common experience is usually caused by an age-related increase in prostate size, called *benign prostatic hypertrophy (BPH)*. Although it is not a "disease" as much as one of the predictable patterns in the biology of a man's life, it can produce symptoms or complications serious enough to require medical attention. Because it occurs in most men as they age, BPH could be called a normal effect of aging. It can produce disturbing symptoms and serious medical complications, however. Benign prostatic hypertrophy is the most common benign tumor found in men and will produce symptoms in the majority of men who live longer than fifty years.

A man who lives eighty years has about an 80 percent chance of having symptoms from BPH and a 30 percent chance of needing surgery. Since these statistics include men prior to the availability of drug therapy, the current likelihood that a man will have surgery may be somewhat less. At age fifty-five, 25 percent of men notice slowing of the urinary stream, while at seventy-five years of age over half of all men experience this problem. A recent study showed that 13 percent of men in their forties had moderate to severe symptoms of BPH, while 28 percent of men over seventy had symptoms of the same severity.

Because of its prevalence, treatment for BPH consumes a considerable amount of resources. About four hundred thousand surgical procedures for BPH are done yearly, making it one of the most

FIGURE 5-1
BPH (Benign Prostate Hypertrophy)

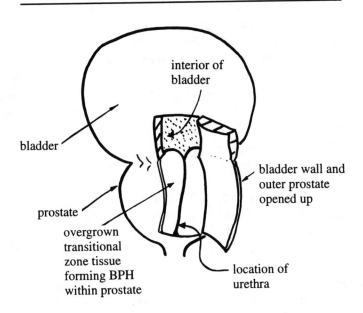

common operations in the United States. It is second after cataract surgery as the most common operation performed, with a total cost of $3 to $4 billion per year in the United States alone.

Because of where the prostate is located, we can see how enlargement may affect the flow of urine from the bladder. This interference is the real problem caused by BPH, as the growth itself is benign. Understanding *obstruction* of the bladder is the key to understanding the various therapies available when BPH causes symptoms. A discussion of drug treatment for BPH requires a brief digression into prostate structure and growth.

WHAT IS BENIGN PROSTATIC HYPERTROPHY?

Many patients have been told they have ''prostate enlargement''—a very common finding on examination. When it is caused by BPH, enlargement is due to growth of a certain part of the prostate in a nonmalignant fashion. *Benign* can mean innocuous or nonthreatening, but in the medical sense the word characterizes a certain type of growth or cell proliferation. The cell multiplication that causes BPH is regulated; expansion of enlarging tissue is limited to the prostate. By comparison, in malignant cell proliferation, such as prostate cancer, there are fewer controls on cellular growth; dividing cells no longer respond to the complex regulatory symptoms that subordinate individual cell activity to the overall good of the organism.

Immediately around the urethra as it leaves the bladder and enters the prostate gland is a region of smooth muscle. This muscle functions as a mechanism to close the upper part of the prostatic urethra during ejaculation and ensures that the semen is forced down the channel and out of the body rather than back into the bladder. This muscle layer will be important as we discuss treatment of BPH, for there are drugs that act selectively to relax and open the channel within this area. Within the muscle are a series of glandular chambers, known by their proximity to the urethra as *periurethral glands.* This group of glands and their drainage ducts make up the *transition zone* of the prostate, which is the area where BPH originates.

The result of transitional zone overgrowth into a benign tumor, or *adenoma,* is the alteration of upper urethral anatomy. Because the periurethral glands of the transitional zone are immediately adjacent to the urethra, their growth results in a growing mass of tissue (BPH) that compresses the wall of the urethra inward (see figure 1–6). This is like an expanding doughnut: as the dough rises, the doughnut hole gets smaller and smaller. Reduction in urine flow is due in part to the squeezing effect of the BPH on the urethra, which interferes with urethral function in other ways as well. To initiate urination, the upper or prostatic urethra must be able to relax, dilate slightly, and change its shape from a closed tube to a funnel (see figure 2–1). To the extent that BPH surrounding the urethra alters its flexibility and elasticity, it acts to inhibit the normal process of urination.

Benign prostatic hypertrophy is glandular overgrowth within the prostate that alters upper urethral anatomy and produces symptoms by interfering with normal urination. The glandular and connective tissue overgrowth in the transition zone of the prostate takes place in identifiable regions of the prostate, producing different "shapes" of BPH. In *lateral lobe enlargement,* paired masses of BPH press in from either side of the urethra. It is primarily the lateral lobes that are felt by the doctor during the digital rectal exam. In some cases, BPH grows more in the middle of the urethra and protrudes upward into the bladder. This condition, called *median lobe hypertrophy,* often produces more obstruction than the lateral lobe pattern of growth. A third pattern, *trilobar hypertrophy,* is present when lateral and median lobe enlargement both occur.

In all cases of BPH, the enlarging masses of transitional zone

FIGURE 5-2
Varieties of BPH

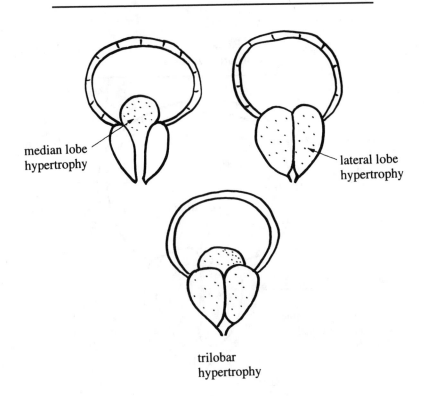

median lobe hypertrophy

lateral lobe hypertrophy

trilobar hypertrophy

overgrowth not only compress the urethra inward, but push the other parts of the prostate outward.

As the inner areas of BPH within the prostate expand, the peripheral parts of the prostate are stretched out into a thin shell. This shell is named the *surgical capsule* of the prostate, because in operations to relieve blockage, the central part of the gland is shelled out of this layer, which remains in the patient after surgery. As we will see later, this peripheral tissue (even if it is stretched out) is where cancers form. That means that after "prostate removal" for BPH, a man can still develop prostate cancer. The surgical capsule is to be distinguished from the *true capsule* of the prostate, which is the thin connective tissue and muscle layer surrounding the glandular tissue within the prostate. This layer is important in containing the spread of prostate cancer and may also contribute to symptoms of obstruction in patients with BPH.

FIGURE 5-3
Prostate Capsules

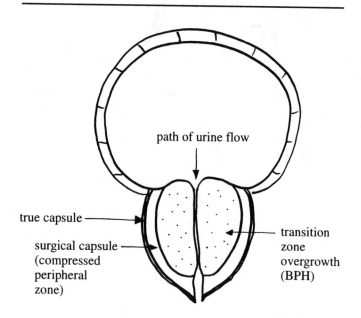

IS BPH MERELY THE OVERABUNDANCE
OF NORMAL PROSTATE TISSUE?

Under the microscope, the appearance of BPH is somewhat different from normal prostate tissue. BPH forms cell-lined spaces suggestive of normal prostate glands, but there are differences. In BPH, the gland spaces are often dilated and filled with secretions that cannot escape for lack of a well-defined duct system. In addition to differences in the way cells are arranged, BPH contains dense noncellular areas where muscle and connective tissue are present. Glands and this connective tissue, or *stroma,* form the two chief components of BPH.

FIGURE 5-4
Microscopic View of BPH

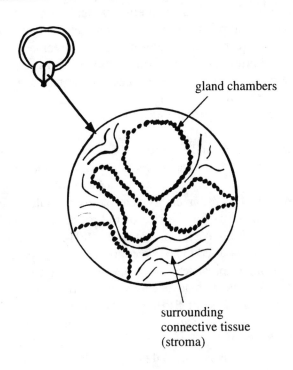

gland chambers

surrounding
connective tissue
(stroma)

Other changes that result from abnormal growth patterns can be seen in BPH tissue. *Infarction* is the death of tissue due to lack of blood supply. Areas of healed infarction are seen in about 25 percent of BPH specimens removed at surgery and may reflect abnormal or marginal blood supply to the overgrowing glands. Areas of infection or inflammation are also quite common in BPH.

WHAT CAUSES BPH?

This question has become the focus of increasingly sophisticated research, as identification of the cause(s) of BPH could conceivably lead to prevention or to more effective therapies. Currently, we do not know the complete story on the origination of BPH, but many of the subplots are being assembled. Most likely, several factors are involved. Young men do not develop BPH, nor do men who lack secretion of the male sex hormone, *testosterone*. Clearly, the cause of BPH involves aging and some effect of male sex hormones.

Studies done on men undergoing prostate removal have shown a relationship between the degree of prostate enlargement and blood levels of sex hormones. In men, small amounts of *estrogen* as well as testosterone are present in the blood. While testosterone levels gradually decline with advancing years, men with larger amounts of BPH seem to have larger amounts of testosterone and estrogen than men with little or no BPH.

Between ages fifty and seventy, BPH grows rapidly enough to double the size of the tumor every ten years. In men older than seventy, the growth rate goes down by a factor of ten.

At these growth rates, an eighty-year-old man would have to live another hundred years for the size of the prostate to double. This observation may help to explain that while BPH is very common in aging men, only about 20 to 30 percent of men will eventually need surgery. Slowing of prostate growth may reflect gradually declining levels of testosterone with advancing years. Hormones in the bloodstream are not the cause of BPH, but a certain amount of hormone is necessary for BPH to occur. Testosterone is converted to a related substance, *dihydrotestosterone,* by an enzyme known as *5-alpha reductase.* An enzyme is a special protein that serves as a catalyst in

Figure 5-5
Growth Rate of BPH

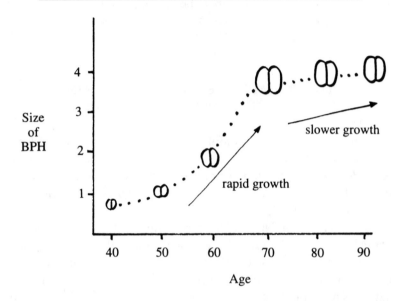

order to speed up a chemical reaction. The effects of the hormone within the prostate cell are actually caused not by testosterone but by its derivative, dihydrotestosterone. One of the medicines used in the treatment of BPH, finasteride (Proscar,[R] Merck), inhibits 5-alpha reductase, preventing the conversion of free testosterone from the bloodstream into its active derivative, dihydrotestosterone. This medication reduces the necessary hormone support required for BPH without changing the testosterone levels in the bloodstream.

As we think back to our brief tour of cell biology in chapter 1, it seems that cell growth within a tissue would be revealed by increasing rates of DNA synthesis. This is the stuff *chromosomes* are made of, and every cell needs a set. Increasing numbers of cells require production of new chromosomes—a phenomenon measurable as increased rates of DNA synthesis. Laboratory studies have shown that BPH is *not* associated with increased rates of DNA synthesis above the levels of normal tissue. The size of a tissue, or collection of cells, is determined not only by how many new cells are made but also by how many old cells die out. Our population would increase dramatically without increased birth rates if our elders stopped dying. The same situation appears to be taking place in BPH—the cell death rate seems to be reduced, which increases prostate size without increasing the rate of cell multiplication.

WHAT REGULATES THE BALANCE BETWEEN CELL MULTIPLICATION AND CELL DEATH?

Unfortunately, there's no simple answer. In some ways, BPH repeats a process that is first seen as the male embryo develops, then again reappears at the time of puberty. This is the growth outward of glands from the urethra into the surrounding connective tissue to form the prostate.

Studies have shown that the surrounding connective tissue, or stroma, is required in order for prostate gland cells to multiply and enlarge. There appears to be some regulatory interaction between these two components that is necessary for glandular growth. Perhaps this mechanism is responsive to other factors that come and go during the span of a man's life.

The overgrowth of tissue in a man with BPH suggests that the embryonic process of prostate formation has been turned on again, after a long stable period extending from his puberty to late middle age. Perhaps some "biological brake" is applied at the end of adolescence to the formative interaction between prostate glands and their surrounding stroma. Something that happens as we get older, working in the presence of a changing hormonal environment, may allow this brake to start slipping. When that happens, the balance of cell growth and cell death is altered, and the prostate gets bigger.

THE EFFECTS OF OBSTRUCTION ON THE URINARY TRACT

Benign prostatic hypertrophy itself is a benign growth that will not spread or cause ill effects in the individual. Its presence is important only when its growth alters lower urinary tract anatomy enough to interfere with the normal process of voiding. All symptoms and complications of BPH are directly traceable to the process of lower urinary tract obstruction. Knowing how the enlarged prostate encircles and squeezes down on the urethra, we can easily see how blockage can occur.

Urologists usually refer to the blockage produced by the squeezing of overgrown glands on the urethra as *static obstruction*. It is due to the constant pressure of BPH and its effects in preventing opening of the urethra during voiding. The prostate capsule, smooth muscle around the upper urethra, and muscle fibers within the prostatic connective tissue are also potentially obstructive. The effects of these structures in preventing the free flow of urine is termed *dynamic obstruction*. This is not the constant pressure of overgrown tissue bulk; it is due to active squeezing of the urethra by contracting muscle.

The distinction between these two types of obstruction becomes important when we talk about drug therapy for prostate blockage. Different medications affect static and dynamic components. One study has shown that enlarged prostates causing troublesome symptoms contain more connective tissue and muscle than enlarged prostates that cause no symptoms. In another study, drugs used selectively to relax the muscle constituting the ''dynamic'' component of BPH dramatically lowered the pressure within the urethra.

To understand obstruction of the lower urinary tract, we need to be reminded of the bladder's function. Basically it has two: (1) to store urine until a convenient time comes along, and (2) to empty itself completely during the process of urination. Nearly all of the BPH symptoms that bring men into doctors' offices can be traced to disturbance in these two functions.

BLADDER EMPTYING

In order for the bladder to empty itself freely, two conditions are required: (1) The urethra or exit tube must not be blocked, and (2) the bladder must squeeze down on the urine and pump it out. Problems in either of these areas can cause major problems with urination. BPH produces both static and dynamic obstruction, but it can also lead to abnormalities in the function of the bladder muscle. The changes produced by blockage of urinary outflow can gradually affect the "pump" function of the bladder; to say that BPH only "narrows down the pipes" is an oversimplification.

The bladder is a hollow muscle that in normal circumstances can raise its internal pressure by contracting. Urination should completely empty the bladder. With increasing blockage of urine, this may be more difficult to accomplish. One measure of obstruction is the amount of urine left in the bladder, or *residual urine*, following urination (see figure 2–3). Residual urine is not always due to obstruction, but significant obstruction usually produces some residual urine.

Normal voiding is a balance between resistance to flow (blockage) and the degree of pressure applied by the bladder. Blockage of urinary flow can be overcome to some degree by increasing the pressure within the bladder. If the bladder "pumps" harder through a restricted channel, it can keep up with its job of emptying. This compensation by the bladder takes the form of muscle building. As the outflow of urine becomes more restricted the bladder becomes more muscular and generates high pressure by squeezing harder. Usually the bladder is thin-walled and smooth. Increase in muscularity produces thickening of the bladder wall and an irregular or ribbed appearance of the inner lining, called *trabeculation*. Thickening of the bladder and trabeculation are both fairly reliable signs of bladder obstruction.

These changes take several years to develop. Exactly how the bladder "feels" blockage and subsequently increases its muscle mass is not known. If the amount of obstruction reaches a steady point or declines over time, the increased strength of the bladder establishes a new balance between blockage and pressure, and bladder emptying may continue fairly effectively. This is called *compensated obstruction*. Increased bladder muscularity stiffens the bladder and causes problems, so compensated obstruction may result in bladder emptying at the price of bothersome symptoms.

If obstruction increases over time, the ability of the bladder to compensate with increased squeezing is gradually overcome. At some point, the bladder fails to keep up with the blockage. This

FIGURE 5-6
Effect of Blockage on Bladder Muscle

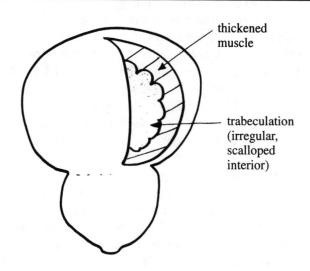

thickened
muscle

trabeculation
(irregular,
scalloped
interior)

causes the accumulation of more and more residual urine as the
bladder muscle loses its fight with blockage. In time, voiding
achieves only a partial reduction in the amount of urine in the
bladder. In this situation, the bladder gradually becomes more
stretched out, holding increased amounts of urine; voiding only
"takes the top off." Over years this situation can cause permanent
loss of bladder contraction. The bladder becomes a floppy sack that
can be emptied only by "pushing" with the abdominal muscles.

STORAGE WITHIN THE BLADDER

In addition to the effects obstructive BPH has on bladder emptying,
the changes it produces in the bladder wall may also interfere with
its ability to store urine.

Storage is the ability to contain urine at low pressures. As the
kidney produces urine, the ability of the bladder to gradually fill up

without generating much pressure is a consequence of passive relaxation in its muscular walls. Bladder muscle must contract and work as a pump to empty urine during the act of voiding, as well as expand passively and stretch out under low pressure in the process of storing urine. Normally, tension within the bladder muscle occurs when the bladder is full and conditions are proper to proceed with voiding. For the bladder to accommodate or store urine comfortably, the muscle must be able to relax without contraction. *Distensibility* of the bladder wall is the ability to expand "loosely." Normal urinary tract function requires that the bladder act both as a strong muscle for voiding and as a loose expandable reservoir.

Sudden increase in the tension of the bladder wall produces an uncomfortable feeling of urgency—a strong desire to void. Avoidance of this annoying symptom is not the only reason the bladder must accommodate urine at low pressure, however. The kidneys act as a filtration system to rid the bloodstream of unwanted waste products. Although the manner by which this is accomplished is extremely sophisticated, one simple prerequisite for normal filtra-

FIGURE 5-7
Distensibility of the Bladder

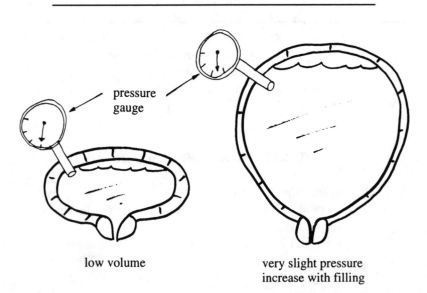

pressure gauge

low volume

very slight pressure increase with filling

tion is the absence of back pressure. The kidney cannot function effectively as a filter when its output is subject to increased pressures. That means that the drainage tube from the kidney to the bladder (the ureter) must be able to carry urine away from the kidney under very low pressure. In order for urine to travel freely from the ureter to the bladder, the pressure in the ureter must be above the pressure in the bladder. If the bladder is unable to store urine at low pressure, the ureter will be unable to transport urine from the kidney, which means the pressure at the "output end" of the kidney filters will rise. This will lead to ineffective filtration function of the kidney and, in time, kidney failure. This primary function of the urinary system depends on the ability of the bladder to fill up easily without increases in its internal pressure.

Adaptive changes in the muscular wall of the bladder that occur in response to the obstruction caused by BPH can reduce the flexibility of the bladder wall in several ways. The thickened, or *hypertrophied,* bladder is stiffer than a normal bladder, so its walls pull tight and we feel "fuller" at lower urinary volumes. Also, the highly muscular bladder is "on its own" more than the normal bladder under strict nerve control. The result of this independent activity of overgrown bladder muscle is that the bladder may begin to contract involuntarily when it gets full, producing a sense of urgency to urinate suddenly. With long-standing overstretching of a bladder in response to blockage and inability to empty, its walls may gradually be replaced with increased quantities of *collagen.* This is a connective tissue protein found in scar tissue, which lacks the ability to contract like muscle. The end result is a baggy, floppy, overstretched bladder that can't empty well even when the blockage is relieved.

WHAT ARE THE COMPLICATIONS OF BLADDER OBSTRUCTION?

The most common cause of bladder obstruction is BPH, although other causes may lead to the same complications as prostate enlargement. For example, a *urethral stricture* (a scarred, narrowed area), or *neurological paralysis* of the bladder could produce any of the problems described here.

FIGURE 5-8
Abnormal Bladder Wall

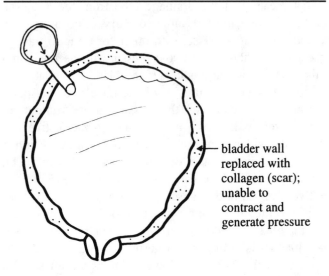

bladder wall
replaced with
collagen (scar);
unable to
contract and
generate pressure

Urinary retention is the inability to empty the bladder. Acute retention is a painful condition in which urination becomes completely impossible and the bladder becomes unbearably full. It almost always requires the placement of a catheter for relief. *Chronic retention* can occur despite the ability to urinate. It is the buildup of urine in the bladder that is periodically reduced by voiding out a small amount, leaving a large amount of *residual urine* that is indefinitely retained in the bladder (see figure 2–3).

Periodic complete emptying is one way to keep the bladder free of infection. Urine is a reasonably good medium for the growth of microorganisms, and if invading bacteria are not flushed out during voiding, infection is more likely. Add to this the distorted glandular overgrowth in BPH that may harbor bacteria, and you can see how urinary tract infection is more common in men with blockage due to BPH. When this occurs with a severe episode of acute retention, the bacteria may enter the bloodstream. The result is *bacteremia,* or *sepsis,* which is a potentially fatal complication of BPH.

Regular emptying of the bladder prevents the minute quantities of dissolved minerals in the urine from building up and forming stones. *Bladder stones* are hard mineral deposits that can range from pea size to baseball size. They usually occur in patients with some element of bladder obstruction, although they may be seen more commonly in patients with gout, when abnormal quantities of uric acid are present in the urine. This substance can contribute to the formation of stones.

The buildup of pressure caused by retention may eventually overcome the one-way valve located where the ureter empties into the bladder. When operating normally, this valve allows the urine from the kidney to enter the bladder after it traverses the ureter, but prevents the increased pressure within the bladder that occurs during voiding from pushing urine back up the ureter. Bladder obstruction

FIGURE 5-9
Other Causes of Difficult Urination

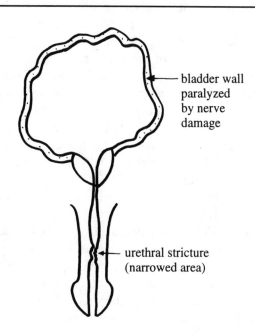

bladder wall
paralyzed
by nerve
damage

urethral stricture
(narrowed area)

from BPH may produce *reflux,* or the abnormal flow of urine up the ureter during urination. This can transmit infection up into the kidney and produce a much more serious urinary tract infection. When reflux accompanies long-standing obstruction, it may transmit dangerously high bladder pressures back into the kidneys' sensitive filtration mechanism.

Renal failure, or the loss of filtering capacity of the kidneys, is the most feared complication of bladder obstruction. When the blockage is properly relieved, it is usually reversible. If renal failure does not respond to relief of obstruction and is not treated, it will cause fatal shifts in the body's chemical balances within about a week. Treatment of renal failure that is unresponsive to relief of obstruction requires *dialysis.* In this process, the bloodstream must be artificially cleaned of waste products by a dialysis machine. It is an arduous medical undertaking, requiring hours of treatment every week, and is associated with its own set of serious complications.

Benign prostatic hypertrophy may also cause *blood in the urine* from a network of fragile varicose (dilated) veins lining the prostatic part of the urethra. If it occurs regularly or results in so much bleeding that clots form in the bladder and impair voiding *(clot retention),* prostate surgery may be necessary.

Structural abnormalities of the bladder can be caused by long-standing blockage. In some cases, the high pressures generated in the obstructed bladder may cause "blowouts" of the bladder lining. These bubble-like pockets are formed when a weak area in the bladder wall allows the inner lining to be pushed out by high internal pressures. The result is a *bladder diverticulum,* which is an outpouching of the bladder lining that usually has no muscle wall and will not empty well with urination. In fact, when the muscle-coated bladder contracts during urination, it pushes urine into this thin wall pocket and enlarges it.

Severe long-standing obstruction may cause the muscular wall of the bladder to undergo structural changes. Collagen, scar tissue that lacks actively working muscle, may build up in the bladder wall, producing a floppy or weak bladder that is more akin to a leather bag than to a living, contracting, muscular organ. This weak, or *atonic,* bladder is often said to represent *myogenic* (muscle-based) *failure,*

FIGURE 5-10
Bladder Diverticula

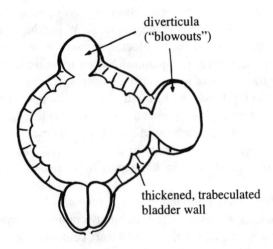

diverticula
("blowouts")

thickened, trabeculated
bladder wall

distinguishing it from the other cause of a weak bladder, *neurogenic failure.* A neurogenic bladder loses its strength when the nerve connections to the bladder are altered (see figure 5–9).

WHAT ARE THE SYMPTOMS OF BLOCKAGE?

We may be able to accept that advancing years slow the stream, but if urine dribbles straight down onto your shoe rather than into the toilet, there may be problems worth investigating. When BPH becomes more obstructive, or if the muscle power of the bladder begins to give out, the stream may slow to the point where patients become irritated by the prolonged time to void. They may feel that they have to stand (or sit) for several minutes to allow the slow stream to empty the bladder. *Hesitancy* (delay in starting the stream), *intermittency* (spontaneous starting and stopping of the stream), or a sensation of *incomplete emptying* after urination may also develop with increasing obstruction. As we reviewed in chapter 2, these symptoms can be produced by a reduction in bladder pressure due to muscle failure, just as they can occur when blockage is present. Diabetics, for instance, may develop muscle weakness in the bladder partly as a result of neurologic difficulties in sensing bladder fullness. In someone with this condition, a relatively mild degree of BPH may produce more severe symptoms. When the bladder can't squeeze normally, or when the blockage is so severe that it impairs emptying, patients may complain of a need to strain to urinate.

Urinary *frequency* is produced when the stiff, muscular bladder begins to pull tight and feel full with smaller amounts of urine. The overactive nature of this "pumped-up" muscle can result in sudden bladder contractions, which cause a feeling of *urgency*. As described in chapter 2, getting up too many times at night is a classic symptom of obstructive BPH, due in large part to increased bladder wall stiffness.

When the muscle contraction that is responsible for overcoming obstruction fails, the bladder fails to empty completely with voiding. This produces residual urine, which can contribute to frequency: Small amounts of urine must be pushed out frequently to reduce the discomfort of a bladder that seems to feel persistently full. Patients who are on the verge of *urinary retention,* the painful condition of being full but unable to void, often complain that they are compelled to void small amounts every ten to fifteen minutes. They can't empty the bladder but try to "take the pressure off" every time the bladder starts to feel full. In this situation, *overflow incontinence* may result. A bladder that is overfilled to begin with may involuntarily leak as the kidneys secrete more urine. This usually occurs at night when muscle control relaxes: *nighttime incontinence,* or *enuresis.*

CAN SERIOUS BLOCKAGE OCCUR WITHOUT SYMPTOMS?

Occasionally, during evaluation of a man with an "abdominal tumor," or dramatic increase in abdominal girth, an overdistended bladder is found. The abdominal mass may shrink when a catheter is inserted, and a quart or two of urine is taken out.

Fortunately, such *silent prostatism* is rare. The gradual failure of bladder muscle to overcome obstruction produces a steady increase in its capacity. If symptoms are absent, the inability to empty may go undetected until the bladder becomes visibly protuberant or other complications occur.

EVALUATION AND TESTING FOR BPH

Evaluation starts with a review of all pertinent symptoms and is followed by a physical examination. When symptoms suggest the possibility of general illness from bladder obstruction, the heart, lungs, and blood pressure are examined for signs of kidney damage or secondary cardiac effects. Usually the examination is confined to the abdomen, genitalia, and rectum.

Tenderness over the kidneys can indicate infection. The abdomen is examined for evidence of bladder distention. This is found by feeling for a firm rounded mass just above the pubic bone or gently tapping this area and listening to the sound. Normally you can hear a hollow sound when you tap over the intestines, which contain a lot of air. If the intestines are pushed away by a bladder distended by urine, a more dull or solid sound is heard. This technique of *percussion* was adapted by early physicians from wine merchants, who could tap on a cask and know where the fluid level was. At the time of genital examination, the testes are checked for tenderness. Urinary tract infection due to obstruction in a man with BPH may travel down the genital duct (vas deferens) and cause *epididymitis* (see figure 1–7). The groin regions are examined for weakness, as continually pushing and straining to urinate can predispose patients with severe BPH to have a *hernia* (weakness and breakdown of the abdominal wall and protrusion of the viscera). Conversely, patients with a hernia should be evaluated for BPH. If they are obstructed and the blockage is not relieved at the time the hernia is repaired, there is a higher chance that the surgical repair will eventually break down.

In most routine cases of prostatism, the rectal exam is the most invasive test required. The size of the prostate can be estimated, although size as determined on a digital rectal exam does not always correlate closely with the degree of obstruction present. For example, a man with a badly obstructed bladder outlet due to median lobe enlargement may have a small and innocuous-feeling prostate gland as revealed by rectal exam. The rectal exam is also mandatory in patients with symptoms of obstruction for the detection of cancer. Pressure within the prostate by an enlarging tumor may cause urinary symptoms, although it is important to emphasize that many patients with cancer have no initial urinary symptoms.

IN THE LABORATORY

Laboratory tests are not necessary to confirm the diagnosis of BPH, as it is not really a disease. Rather, there are ways to determine what impact the obstruction caused by BPH has on the patient. Fortunately, not many are tests required to identify the complications of BPH. A urinalysis is done in men suspected of prostatism to rule out secondary infection. It may also be helpful to identify microscopic blood in the urine, which can lead to the diagnosis of complications such as bladder stones.

The prostate-specific antigen test, or PSA, should be done in all men who are being evaluated for prostate disorder. Some men who develop symptoms from prostate cancer have a prostate that feels like BPH during exam, without lumps or hard spots. The PSA can be instrumental in allowing the diagnosis of cancer to be made as early as possible.

The only other blood test frequently used is serum creatinine, as described in chapter 3. This is a measure of the filtration function of the kidney and helps to identify patients who are in danger of kidney malfunction because of obstruction. Generally it is not necessary to test for serum creatinine unless there is other evidence of fairly severe obstruction such as large residual amounts of urine or acute retention of urine.

OTHER STUDIES

Not too long ago it was necessary to catheterize a bladder to measure residual urine present after voiding. Now, ultrasound is very effective in measuring the size of the bladder while allowing a reasonably accurate calculation of bladder volume. Ultrasound can also be used to detect problems higher in the urinary tract, dilation of the kidney, or *hydronephrosis* due to blockage (see figure 3–7). The intravenous pyelogram permits the entire urinary tract to be examined and the degree of bladder emptying to be determined, but it requires X-ray exposure and the use of intravenous X-ray dye. It is usually reserved for patients with BPH who also have microscopic blood in the urine or other evidence of possible structural abnormalities.

Measurement of urinary stream velocity, or *uroflometry,* is helpful in evaluating patients with BPH. It is a noninvasive test that requires the patient to come in for testing with a full bladder and to void into a specially monitored commode. For this test to be accurate, the patient must void 150 milliliters or more. Maximum flow rates of less than 10 milliliters per second usually suggest blockage. Men with maximum flow rates of greater than 15 milliliters per second generally are not obstructed. (Seven or eight percent of these men can be blocked, but are able to flow at good rates due to dramatic compensatory muscle buildup of the bladder.)

For more severe cases, such as patients with suspected BPH who have other problems that might also affect bladder emptying, more complicated *urodynamic tests* can be done. These tests allow urine flow to be measured simultaneously with bladder pressures, and obstruction to be diagnosed most precisely. Not all cases of low flow are due to blockage; they may be due to bladder disorders that cause ineffectively low pressures. Very few men with BPH require this type of testing.

Cystoscopy allows visual inspection of the prostate (see figure 3–8). Although it can be accomplished in the doctor's office with the patient under local anesthesia, it is uncomfortable and can cause infection, bleeding, or irritation of the urethra. In some cases when surgery is planned, it may be required to determine the best operative approach. Occasionally, it is used to confirm the presence of bladder stones when they are suspected or to evaluate the urinary tract carefully when microscopic blood has been found.

The majority of men with prostatism can be adequately evaluated with a physical exam, urinalysis, PSA, and—if the symptoms are bothersome—a uroflow test. When symptoms are severe or the uroflow gives flow rates of less than 10, measurement of post-void residual urine by ultrasound is helpful. It is not usually necessary to check kidney function with a serum creatinine unless the residual volume is over 100 milliliters or the patient has some other condition that could affect kidney function.

TREATMENT OF BPH

A few years ago, this section would have been shorter, starting and ending with surgery. At that time, symptoms of BPH were either mild enough to live with or severe enough to warrant surgery.

The proper management for patients with catheter dependency, kidney damage, or bladder stones hasn't changed since then; surgery is still required and is detailed in chapter 7. Patients with bothersome symptoms without these complications, however, now have an increased choice of new therapies. Selecting the one most appropriate for a single individual requires personal consultation with the doctor. This is a good place to reemphasize that managing BPH is not the same as treating a disease. The treatment of BPH is really the treatment of its symptoms and complications, which vary in each individual. When illness is caused by a clearly defined "villain," such as infectious bacteria, treatment is fairly standardized for all. When symptoms occur without illness, treatment must be more individually tailored. Moreover, since most men over fifty have some symptoms of BPH, the most important question is who should be treated and who can safely be reassured and monitored without treatment.

In this expanding era of multiple alternative therapies, the indications for treatment do not rely solely on the patient's condition. They also depend on the risks, expense, impact, and complications of the specific treatment under consideration. For example, patients for whom drug therapy has been properly recommended may not necessarily be candidates for surgery. Cases that warrant the risks of medication may not be severe enough to warrant the risks of surgery. Conversely, the severely obstructed individual with bladder stones and secondary infection may never get better with medicines alone and should be treated surgically without delay.

With the wide range of treatment options now available, it is important to realize that some methods are more proven than others and that follow-up studies detailing results are not uniform from method to method.

THE NATURAL HISTORY OF BPH—
WHAT HAPPENS WITHOUT TREATMENT

Patients with modest symptoms would favor treatment if they knew things would eventually get worse as time passed, and would probably forgo treatment if the future held stabilization or improvement. Unfortunately, the course of an individual's symptoms are not predictable, although statistics for groups of men have been collected regarding the natural history of prostatism—its natural course when untreated. In studies of men observed without treatment, one-third to two-thirds improved over approximately five years. The number of patients who worsened and eventually needed surgery ranged from 10 to 45 percent. In another study of men found by rectal examination to have an enlarged prostate, those who also complained of a feeling of incomplete emptying and a weakened urinary stream had a 38 percent chance of eventually needing surgery.

REASONS TO TREAT BPH

Many patients with prostatism want treatment simply to alleviate certain symptoms. There is nothing wrong with this as long as the doctor has reviewed the various risks of treatment, and both doctor and patient are in agreement that the magnitude of the problem outweighs the possible risks of the treatment.

In some cases, there may be less choice in the decision making. Patients who need catheter placement for inability to void, and have failed to void when the catheter has been removed after an adequate period of time, require surgery. If they are extremely elderly or fragile, some may wish to live their lives with the catheter rather than taking the risks of surgery. New surgical methods, like *laser prostatectomy* (see chapter 7) may be safe enough to use in patients who are too frail for conventional surgery. Other compelling reasons to undergo surgery for BPH are the accumulation of substantial amounts of residual urine, deterioration of kidney function, persistent urinary infection, *overflow incontinence,* or bladder stones. Men with BPH may also suffer recurring urinary tract bleeding severe enough to require surgery, but this condition is rare.

MEDICAL TREATMENT OF BPH

Medication can be helpful in alleviating many of the symptoms of BPH. Currently, two classes of drugs are available for the treatment of prostatism. One acts upon the conversion of male hormone within the prostate cells, and the other relaxes the muscle in and around the prostate. These two groups of drugs correspond to the two components of blockage produced by the prostate, described previously. *Static obstruction* is the mechanical blockage produced by the en-

FIGURE 5-11
Static and Dynamic Resistance to Flow

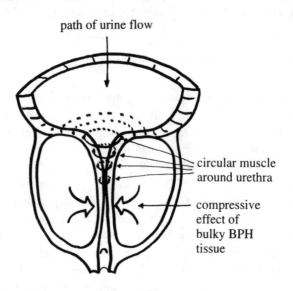

path of urine flow

circular muscle
around urethra

compressive
effect of
bulky BPH
tissue

larged mass of prostate tissue and is composed largely of overgrown glands. *Dynamic obstruction* is the restriction of urine flow through the prostatic urethra due to the squeezing effect of muscle fibers within and surrounding the prostate. These are not the type of muscles that are under voluntary control.

Only one medication currently available, Proscar® (finasteride, Merck), is active against static obstruction. It shrinks the prostate by altering the hormone metabolism within the gland. Several drugs are available that affect dynamic obstruction by selective relaxation of prostatic muscle fibers. These are called selective alpha-1 blockers, two of which are Minipress® (prazosin, Pfizer) and Hytrin® (terazosin, Abbott).

SHRINKING THE PROSTATE: THE EFFECT OF HORMONES ON PROSTATE GROWTH

Prostate growth does not occur in boys who lose testosterone production before puberty. Scientific research into some of the reasons for this have led to Proscar®, a drug that can reduce prostate size by interfering with the metabolism of male hormones within prostate cells. Testosterone affects libido, sexual function, muscular development, metabolism, and red blood cell production. Drugs that stop testosterone production are available but have too many undesirable side effects to be used routinely in healthy men with symptoms of BPH only. They are employed successfully in the control of prostate cancer and will be discussed further in chapter 6.

Testosterone affects prostate cell metabolism by causing special proteins to bind to the DNA within the cell nucleus and direct cell growth. It turns out that over 90 percent of the hormone activity within the prostate cell comes not from testosterone but from its derivative, dihydrotestosterone. Moreover, the protein that binds to DNA and causes cell growth requires dihydrotestosterone, not testosterone. As we have reviewed, 5-alpha reductase is the enzyme responsible for converting testosterone into this active derivative.

Previous research suggested that a possible way to stop prostate cell growth without changing a man's blood testosterone level would be to block this enzyme conversion step. The enzyme 5-alpha reductase has no other function than the conversion of testosterone, and men who are born with a deficiency of the enzyme have normal life spans.

Laboratory work has shown that a specific 5-alpha reductase inhibitor, Proscar® (finasteride, Merck), was able to reduce the dihydrotestosterone content of the prostate and shrink its overall size. Early clinical studies showed this drug reduced prostate volume 20 to 30 percent, improved urine flow, and reduced symptoms.

OUT OF THE LAB AND INTO THE CLINIC

The safety and effectiveness of Proscar® for the treatment of BPH was evaluated recently in two large studies: a North American group of 895 men and an international group of 750 men. Prostate shrinkage ranged from 19 to 24 percent in treated patients, compared with 3 to 6 percent in patients receiving a placebo. There was considerable variability in the amount of size reduction, however. About 60 percent of men receiving Proscar® experienced significant prostate shrinkage. Men entering this study were found to have a maximal urinary flow rate of about 9.5 milliliters per second before treatment. Although maximal urinary flow rates increased more in treated patients as a group than in those receiving the placebo, only about 30 percent of treated patients had improvement in flow rates above the change seen in patients receiving the placebo.

The symptoms of prostatism (slow stream, frequency, getting up at night, etc.) were evaluated on a scoring system (see table 5–1). The score did not change much following treatment in those patients with minimal symptoms. In patients with severe symptoms, however, the overall symptom score dropped by approximately six to seven points—quite a bit compared with the one-point improvement in patients receiving the placebo. Overall, or "global," improvement was reported in about 60 to 70 percent of treated patients compared with 50 to 60 percent in men receiving the placebo.

Sexual function appears to be sensitive to serum testosterone

TABLE 5-1
American Urological Association Symptom Score

Over the last months how often have you	Not at all	Less than one time in five	Less than half the time	About half the time	More than half the time	Almost always
felt that you have not completely emptied your bladder	0	1	2	3	4	5
have you had to urinate less than 2 hours after emptying	0	1	2	3	4	5
stopped and started several times during urination	0	1	2	3	4	5
found it difficult to postpone urination	0	1	2	3	4	5
had a weak urinary stream	0	1	2	3	4	5
had to push or strain to begin urination	0	1	2	3	4	5
did you most typically get up at night to urinate	not at all	once every 8 hours	once every 4 hours	once every 3 hours	once every 2 hours	at least once every hour
	0	1	2	3	4	5

levels, which are not decreased by therapy with Proscar®. Despite this, a very slight incidence of sexual dysfunction was observed in these studies. Impotence was experienced by 3.7 percent of men receiving Proscar® compared with 1.1 percent in placebo-treated patients. Problems with *libido* (sex drive) and ejaculation were reported about 3 percent of the time by men receiving Proscar® compared with 1.4 percent of the time in those receiving placebo. There were no other significant adverse effects from treatment, although most patients receiving Proscar® experienced a slight reduction in the amount of semen produced during ejaculation.

USE OF PROSCAR®

At this time, there are no data to support the use of Proscar® as a preventive treatment for prostatism. As outlined above, the results seen in men with minimal symptoms are poor. Proscar® should be used when symptoms are moderate to severe, corresponding to seven points or greater on the symptoms score (see table 5–1). Once again, this drug should not be used if urinary obstruction has impaired kidney function or resulted in urinary retention that does not clear up when the catheter is removed. Every patient who is given Proscar® should have a digital rectal exam and a PSA test. Any abnormalities discovered by these tests should be evaluated in the usual manner. Issues regarding the use of this drug in patients with high PSA values are outlined in further detail in chapter 6. In addition to these studies, the measurement of urinary flow rate at the beginning of therapy is helpful as a basis for further comparisons as drug therapy is maintained.

DYNAMIC BLOCKAGE: THE EFFECT OF MUSCLE FIBERS ON URINARY TRACT OBSTRUCTION

While Proscar® emerged from prostate research, a different class of drugs effective against the symptoms of prostatism has come to us from research on high blood pressure. Regulation of muscle tension in the wall of an artery controls the blood pressure: Constriction of the muscle fibers surrounding an artery raises the internal blood pressure, while relaxation of them increases the channel size of the artery, reducing blood pressure. These muscles in the artery wall harbor a *receptor,* or biochemical switching mechanism, called the *alpha-1 receptor.*

We have discussed how the bladder is a hollow muscle and how its contraction is necessary for voiding. We have also described the "dynamic" component of prostate blockage, which is caused by muscle squeezing; paralysis of the muscle fibers in and around the prostate reduces the constriction of the channel by about 40 percent. Blocking all muscle action in the lower urinary tract would open up the channel but paralyze the bladder and make urination difficult. Fortunately, the muscles making up the bladder, and those contributing to blockage, are controlled by different signals. This allows selective "blocking" of the receptors in the muscles surrounding the channel that contribute to urinary obstruction. It turns out that these muscles constituting the dynamic component of urethral block-

FIGURE 5-12
Common Muscle Action in Bladder and Blood Vessels

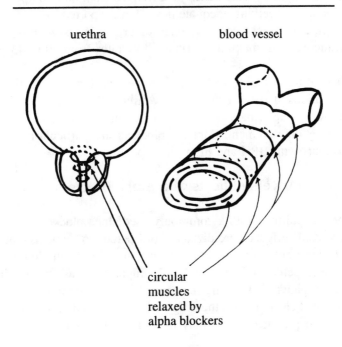

urethra   blood vessel

circular
muscles
relaxed by
alpha blockers

age are under the same control as the muscles surrounding blood vessels—the alpha-1 receptor.

The drugs that block this chemical switching mechanism and prevent internal signals from causing muscle contraction are called *alpha-1 blockers.* These drugs are effective in lowering both blood pressure and the constriction of the prostatic urethra caused by BPH. They were among the first medications useful in the treatment of symptoms due to BPH.

Results with Alpha Blocker Therapy

The beneficial effect of these drugs is dose related: they are unlikely to work at extremely low doses. Increasing dosage means increasing the chance of unwanted side effects, but as we will see, side effects are not usually a problem. At the time of writing, thirty clinical trials of alpha blockers for prostatism have been done, with twenty-seven reporting positive results. The overall likelihood of a patient benefiting from alpha blocker therapy has ranged from 60 to 85 percent. Most patients receiving adequate doses have reported improvement in daytime and nighttime frequency of urination, as well as measured increases in maximum urinary flow rates from 20 to 43 percent.

These drugs should not be used to treat prolonged retention or complications of BPH such as kidney failure. Pretreatment and six-month follow-up urinary flow rates are helpful as objective means of measuring improvement. Alpha-1 blockers are particularly suited for patients with BPH and high blood pressure.

Adverse Effects with Alpha Blockers

In one clinical trial with a commonly used alpha blocker, the most common side effects were dizziness (14 percent of patients), headache (10 percent), weakness (7 percent), and abnormally low blood pressure (2 percent). In another study impotence was reported in 4 percent of patients. A smaller number of patients reported a flu-like reaction that cleared when the drug was discontinued. Since the dose required to produce results may be difficult to predict, it is often necessary for the doctor to gradually *titrate* (adjust) the amount of medication until it is high enough to produce improvement in prostatism but low enough to avoid side effects.

Specific Alpha Blockers

Prazosin (Minipress®, Pfizer) was the first selective alpha-1 blocker used for BPH. In one series, 2 milligrams per day increased peak urinary flow rates by about 60 percent, compared with an increase of 6 percent in the group receiving a placebo. In another study, twenty-five of forty patients who received 3 to 4.5 milligrams per day showed improvement in frequency and flow rates, without adverse effects. Compared with terazosin, prazosin has a shorter duration of effect. This usually makes it necessary to take the medication twice a day.

Terazosin (Hytrin®, Abbott) is the selective alpha-1 blocker that has been most widely studied in the treatment of BPH. Its relatively long-lasting efficacy allows it to be taken in a single daily dose. The best results are obtained in patients who take 5 to 10 milligrams per day. At this level, the overall symptom score tends to decrease by close to 50 percent, and maximum urinary flow rates increase by approximately 42 percent. The adverse effects seen were similar to those described above, and all were reversible by stopping the medication. In long-term studies, patients receiving medication for two years continued to experience good results, showing that the drug effect does not seem to lessen over time.

Combination Therapy

Since finasteride and alpha-1 blockers each affect different components of prostate obstruction, there may be good reason to use them both. Preliminary studies have pointed to an additive effect of alpha blocker and hormone manipulation in combination, but at this writing there have been no controlled trials or firm clinical guidelines for this approach. Common sense suggests that the drugs be started one at a time, in order to show more about a particular patient's response.

TABLE 5–2
BPH Treatments

Treatment	Indications	Side effects	Results	Duration of effects	Risk and complications	Cost
Observation	Mild-moderate symptoms	—	—	—	20–30% chance of progression	$75/year
Medications Proscar®	Bothersome symptoms, (score > 7 on table 5-1), residual urine	Rare reduction in libido	15–20% increase in flow rates, symptom improvement	As long as medication is taken	Effect on PSA may make early cancer detection difficult	$725/year
Alpha blockers (Hytrin®, etc.)	See Proscar	Dizziness, headache, weakness	20–30% increase in flow rates, symptom improvement	See Proscar	Very few	$550/year
Conventional surgery Transurethral resection (TURP)	Urinary retention, bothersome symptoms, bladder stones	Retrograde ejaculation	100% increase in flow rate, symptom improvement in 80–90%	No decrease in flow rate over 7 years; redo rate 13%	Transfusion (4%), Stricture (4%), Incontinence (<1%)	$4,000

Transurethral incision (TUIP)	Bothersome symptoms, small prostate	Possible retrograde ejaculation	50% increase in flow rates, symptom improvement	Slightly less than TURP	Regrowth of prostate structure, transfusions, impotence, all about 1–2%, incontinence <1%	$2,000
Open prostatectomy (suprapubic, retropubic)	Symptoms or retention due to prostate stones	Retrograde ejaculation	Slightly better than TURP	Longer than TURP; redo rate is 4%	About the same as TURP, transfusion about 6–8%	$7,500
New technology Laser ablation	See TURP	Prolonged postoperative catheterization	Similar to TURP	Unknown	Failure to correct retention, prolonged burning and frequency	$2,000
Balloon dilation	See TUIP—cannot have median lobe blockage	Possible retrograde ejaculation	Similar to TUIP	Less than 2 years	Failure to correct retention, bleeding	$1,200
Microwave heating	Moderate symptoms	Unknown	Unknown	Unknown	Unknown	Unknown
Prostate stent	Retention	Unknown	Unknown	Unknown	Persistent pain and/or infection	Unknown

BPH REQUIRES PERSONALIZED DECISION MAKING

Benign prostatic hypertrophy is different in everyone. In some cases it is primarily glandular overgrowth that responds to hormonal manipulation, while in other cases muscle and connective tissue play a greater role in obstruction. The biologic variation in BPH is matched by the spectrum of symptoms and complications experienced by men with aging plumbing. For those with mild symptoms, there is probably no need to offer therapy. Of course, such patients should still be evaluated; as we have seen, dangerous obstruction can occasionally exist with minimal symptoms. In addition, any man with symptoms of obstruction should be screened for prostate cancer.

In the past, many men have tolerated moderate to severe symptoms, wishing to avoid the risks of surgery. We are now fortunate to have reasonably effective medical therapy to offer them. Finally, men with significant complications of BPH or severe symptoms have more alternatives now than ever before. On the basis of technical improvement, accumulated experience, and advances in anesthesia and nursing care, conventional surgery is safe and reliable when it is necessary.

Chapter 6

═══════════

PROSTATE CANCER

Jack Chambers' internist had called me about his abnormal lab test results a couple of days before. To look at Jack you would never suspect anything to be wrong. He appeared to be a healthy sixty-year-old, confident and in excellent physical shape. As he reached over and grasped his wife's hand, I realized she was the prime mover in his being here. "Doctor, isn't the PSA test for prostate cancer?"

I looked from one to the other. "Well, not exactly." My first instinct was to reassure them—things are rarely as bad as imagined. Although one can't come to conclusions without clinical facts, my reaction was not just an insincere effort to prop up their outlook. By the time they see me, most patients have imagined their condition to be as frightening as possible, treatable only by arduous, painful, disfiguring, expensive, and ultimately futile therapies.

I try not to sound like a medical professor. "PSA stands for prostate-specific antigen. It's a chemical produced by prostate cells, so it's present in every man's blood. If the prostate enlarges, the PSA level goes up. If prostate cancer develops, then PSA also increases, usually beyond the growth indicator level. So, an elevated PSA doesn't necessarily mean cancer is present. It does warn us, however, to be suspicious and do a thorough investigation."

Jack had had an ultrasound-guided prostate biopsy, which was negative. In the following eight months he had two more PSA tests, both of which showed abnormal levels, and as I suspected, the result of a repeat biopsy was positive for cancer. Jack's son brought him over to discuss treatment. He seemed anxious to have a moment with me in private. "Doctor, with my father's condition . . . should I be tested?"

The fear of prostate cancer is to men what the fear of breast cancer is to women. Just the word "cancer" is enough to bring concerns about dying into sharp focus. Although most men who are diagnosed with prostate cancer will not die of it, the mere possibility gives a personal perspective to feelings about life that were previously only abstractions. Like breast cancer, prostate cancer raises the fear of loss of sexuality along with anxiety about painful tests or procedures in a particularly sensitive area.

The diagnosis of cancer can precipitate an exhausting foray into a whole series of "what ifs": What if I lose my independence? What if I can't live the retirement I've saved all my life for, and how will this affect those I care for? What if cancer strikes my loved ones, my business associates? What if my health insurance isn't enough? We all dread a condition that reduces our ability to regulate our own lives, putting us into the hands of a team of doctors.

Although prostate cancer occurs later in life, hopefully when we have the maturity to understand our limits and mortality, it does not always stand in direct opposition to dying of old age. Even though prostate cancer is fairly common, death due to this disease occurs in the minority of men who are diagnosed with it. Statistics will not eliminate worry, but learning more about this common problem will dispel the specter of imagined catastrophe. Hope and optimism are precious assets when your health is in question, and knowing the facts about this manageable disease will help you preserve them.

Now that we have dispensed with life and death, on to more important issues—sex. What if I can't satisfy my partner or even perform at all? This imagined scenario and others are the basis for many of the fears men have about prostate cancer. Treatment will certainly interrupt one's sexual schedule, but it will not end your life as a sexually active man. Some patients may require additional treatment or assistance, but *sex continues after prostate cancer therapy for those who desire it.*

Fear can be a good thing when it propels us into action. For many with a diagnosis of prostate cancer, this means reading and research. Making intelligent decisions based on new-found knowledge is not only practical but, a sure-fire antidote to fear. Unfortunately, condensing the available information into something that makes sense can be a big job.

As more medical studies are publicized, the patient may be overwhelmed by information. Turning to a medical library might seem like the answer, but that just makes it worse. There are so many studies published and so many new approaches being tried that even practicing physicians may be hard pressed to separate the good from the bad. Probably more articles have been written about prostate cancer in the last dozen years than in the previous dozen centuries. You may feel lost as you survey this vast swamp of observation and opinions, where tomorrow's advances lie hidden among false assumptions and soon-to-be-forgotten "discoveries."

To navigate this information overload, you will need help. Theory and proposals need to be filtered through experience by one who knows what has been done in the past, what works, what doesn't, and what your needs are. This requires a physician who is well informed and able to communicate effectively.

THE NUMBERS

Prostate cancer is the most common malignancy in men. It is not the most common cause of cancer-related death in men, however, because unlike the leader in this grim category, lung cancer, prostate cancer is not usually lethal. It is projected that in 1994, one hundred sixty-five thousand new cases of prostate cancer will be diagnosed in this country, and thirty-five thousand deaths will occur. An American man has a 10 percent chance of being diagnosed with prostate cancer in his lifetime but only a 2 to 3 percent chance of dying from it. Clearly, many more men live with prostate cancer than die from it.

Prostate cancer has important relationships to race, geography, and age. For example, the incidence of prostate cancer in American black men is up to 80 percent greater than the incidence in American white men. A twenty-five-fold increase in the incidence of prostate cancer was found in black men living in San Francisco, compared with Japanese men in the same city. Japanese men living in Japan have a lower incidence of prostate cancer than those who have emigrated to the United States, and African-American men have a higher incidence of prostate cancer than do blacks living in Africa.

The risk of cancer of the prostate is increased in men with close blood relatives who have developed the disease. While most cases of prostate cancer do not occur in a family pattern, heredity can clearly be a factor in this disorder. The chance of developing prostate cancer is increased two- to three-fold in men whose fathers or brothers have the disease and is increased up to five times normal if two or more close relatives are affected.

Nutrition may play a role in preventing prostate cancers. Research has shown that a diet high in animal fats is associated with a higher incidence of advanced prostate cancer.

Recent reports have indicated that men who have a *vasectomy* may be at increased risk for prostate cancer. The scientific evidence surrounding this issue is conflicting. For this reason, a meeting on this subject was recently held at the National Institutes of Health. It included a large panel of researchers and experts in this field, and their consensus was that current practices regarding vasectomy should continue unchanged. Previous studies have failed to turn up a link between vasectomy and prostate cancer, and there is no known biological reason why there should be such a link. While acknowledging that this question deserves further research, and recommending that men who have undergone vasectomy be examined annually after age fifty for prostate cancer, they emphasized that no form of contraception is without risk.

Prostate cancer is age related, becoming more and more common as men pass fifty. The incidence of this disease increases faster with age than that of any other cancer. Aging men may become ill with prostate cancer, or they may harbor it and never know. This is a good place to introduce the distinction between *histologic cancer* and *clinical cancer.* Histologic refers to cancer that is present on microscope slides made from prostate tissue removed at the time of autopsy. In older men who have died from any of several other illnesses, microscopic areas of the prostate commonly appear cancerous when closely examined. Clinical cancer is present in those patients who develop (or are at risk to develop) symptoms or problems due to prostate cancer. Men found to have histologic prostate cancer at autopsy were usually not affected by or diagnosed with prostate cancer in their lifetimes. Conversely, about a fourth of men found to have clinical cancer will die from it.

This variety in the behavior of prostate cancer has always been appreciated. With increasingly sensitive methods of cancer diagnosis, however, it has drawn more attention to decisions regarding treatment. There was little question that treatment appeared necessary in those patients diagnosed in the past, when a hard enlarging tumor could be felt by examination. There is still no question regarding the need to aggressively treat prostate cancer in a young man. In an elderly man, microscopic cancers may never develop into illness. In this setting, we would have to question the wisdom of treating a patient who wasn't ill with cancer, and who probably never would be. Sixty to 70 percent of all men over eighty are found at autopsy to harbor these microscopic histologic cancers. Certainly, exposing someone to the risks and expense of treatment makes no sense if he is to live a full life and die without any outward sign of prostate cancer.

It seems that prostate cancer appears in two different "forms": an incidental finding at autopsy, or a disease-producing process diagnosed during life. Attempting to explain this dual existence, doctors have developed two theoretical possibilities. The first theory is that two different types of prostate cancer exist: an indolent or innocuous type, and an aggressive or spreading type. Perhaps the process of aging produces the indolent type, whereas something else is responsible for the aggressive variety. The second theory is that there is only one type of prostate cancer, which gets worse as it grows larger. These possibilities both have supporting evidence, but they still are only theories. If we knew the real story, much of the controversy surrounding who should be treated would be eliminated. Fortunately, research offers clinical advice from both proposals. We are beginning to identify which tumor cells are likely to be the aggressive type, and learning that tumors of sufficient size (larger than ½ milliliter in volume) are at increased risk of developing into clinical cancer.

These issues become increasingly important with the "graying" of America. In the 1980s, there were thirty million people older than sixty-five; by the year 2000, this group will increase to forty-five million. Not only will this increase the prevalence of latent prostate cancer, it will produce a growing number of men with clinical prostate cancer that will require appropriate cost and risk-effective management.

WHAT IS CANCER?

Living in a constantly changing environment, our bodies are remarkable in their ability to remain the same. Yes, we age too quickly and never fail to notice the effects, but the components making up our bodies maintain their form day to day, with very little variation.

Over several years, in a process of miraculous complexity, development takes us from a single cell to apparent stability as an adult. The constancy of our biologic structure is only an outward appearance, an illusion of stability enacted by the unseen interplay of millions of cells involved in a complex choreography of division, maturation, and death. The control and regulatory process responsible for this coordination are beyond our understanding, but they link the activities of each individual cell with the overall well-being of the entire organism.

A break in this link may allow cell growth to continue in an unregulated or independent fashion. When the cellular abnormalities that allow a cell to drift free from the enveloping order of the body are inheritable, or passed to the next generation of cells, the growth of abnormal tissue results. When the body's surveillance and containment systems fail and this growth is allowed to persist, cancer results. *Cancer is unauthorized, uncontrolled, and disorganized cell division resulting in the growth of tissue that is foreign to the body's overall plan.*

Cancer cells differ from normal cells by genetic, inheritable alterations in areas of their DNA that direct growth control. The change from a normal cell to a cancer cell is called *malignant transformation.* Laboratory study of these transformed, or cancer, cells has shown that they differ in several ways from normal cells. They will grow in a liquid culture medium, while normal cells require a firm substance to cling to. When cultured upon a surface, they do not show the normal *contact inhibition,* or retardation of cell division, when they grow out and crowd into other surrounding

FIGURE 6-1
Properties of Normal Cells and Cancer Cells

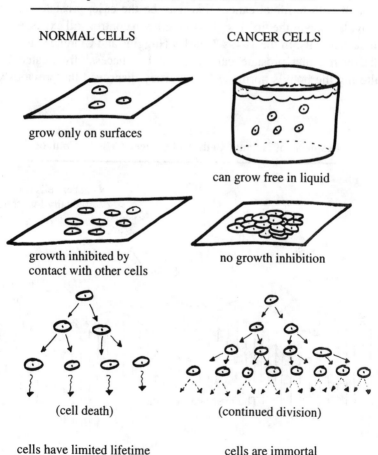

NORMAL CELLS   CANCER CELLS

grow only on surfaces

can grow free in liquid

growth inhibited by
contact with other cells

no growth inhibition

(cell death)   (continued division)

cells have limited lifetime   cells are immortal cells. Finally, these cells are immortal—they just keep on dividing when given sufficient culture medium.

Even with optimal conditions, normal cells in culture have a finite life span. It is easy to understand why cells with these properties could, with continued growth, end up in parts of the body where they don't belong.

Seeing cancer deposits, or *metastases,* throughout the body in patients dying of cancer, early pathologists concluded that the proliferation of cancer cells was totally independent and unresponsive to any of the body's regulatory mechanisms (see figure 2–5). Although with terminal cancer this may be the case, prostate cancer provided one of the first insights that growth control still exists, even in cancer cells. In the 1940s, Charles Huggins and Clarence Hodges discovered that prostate cancer could be successfully treated by altering the body's hormone levels. They disproved the previously

FIGURE 6-2
Response of Normal Cells and Cancer Cells to Control

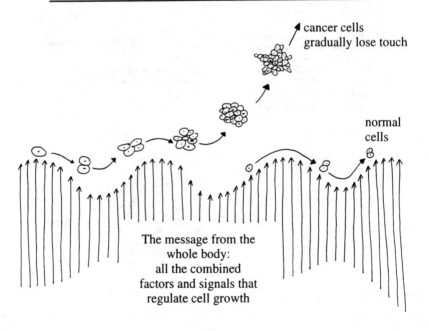

cancer cells
gradually lose touch

normal
cells

The message from the
whole body:
all the combined
factors and signals that
regulate cell growth

held idea that cancer cells were entirely independent of all control mechanisms.

Contemporary research is enlarging our understanding of how complex and multilayered growth control really is. Cancer seems to be more than just a single foul-up in the blueprint for cellular division. For a malignant cancer to occur, it appears that these foul-ups must accumulate over time, gradually compounding each other and steadily increasing the anarchy of cellular behavior.

Normal cells interact with their surrounding environment at the outer wall, or *cell membrane.* By combining with molecular structures in the cell membrane called *receptors,* chemical messages can affect cell growth. This occurs when the chemical messenger sticks to the receptor and causes a chemical reaction in the cell that sends a second message inward to the cell nucleus (see figure 1–11). This secondary signal interacts with the cell's "information bank," or DNA, producing a programmed response of cellular activities. Abnormalities in the DNA segments, or *genes,* that contain the instructions for building and operating this secondary messenger system can cause cancer.

The idea that cancer must involve an inheritable, or transmitted, abnormality in cellular behavior was proved when DNA taken from a human cancer cell was able to transform a normal mouse cell into a cancer cell.

We now know of over one hundred different segments of DNA that cause malignant transformation of a cell. They are of two types: *oncogenes,* which work to increase cell growth, and *tumor suppressor genes,* which act to retard or brake cell growth. Their common attribute is that they affect a cell's ability to control the growth process. These genes, usually involved in the normal process of cell division, can become cancer-causing when mutation or other DNA changes result in increased oncogene activity, decreased tumor suppressor activity, or both.

Apparently, cancer is not caused by a single genetic error in the growth control mechanism. With its onset, this disease seems to put into motion a progressive loss of more and more regulatory functions, an accumulation of genetic mistakes that may require the compounding effect of hundreds of cell generations to become le-

Figure 6-3
Cancer Can Be Created by DNA Transfer

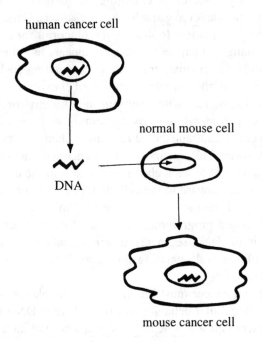

thal. It may take years for a group of cancer cells to gradually acquire the changes that make them capable of metastasizing, or spreading throughout the body.

Because the formation of cancer is a multi-step process, it follows that *cancer initiation* is not sufficient to produce disease. A second set of circumstances or conditions referred to as *cancer promotion* is required. Black men and Japanese men have dramatically different rates of clinical prostate cancer and dramatically different death rates due to prostate cancer. Despite this, the prevalence of histologic cancer found at autopsy in aging black or Japanese men who have died of other causes is remarkably similar. These two groups show a similarity in factors producing *cancer initiation* with aging, but a disparity in those secondary conditions that promote *cancer progression*. Some of these secondary promoting factors are related to environment. This is shown by the difference in clinical cancer between Japanese men in Japan and Japanese-born men living in the United States. The prevalence of histologic cancer is the same in both groups, but clinical prostate cancer is more common in Japanese-Americans.

The cause of cancer is complex. We no longer conceive of this disease as being caused by a single cell's "copier button" becoming stuck, but rather as a property of a growing community of cells that becomes more and more anarchistic as time goes by.

WHAT ARE THE SYMPTOMS OF PROSTATE CANCER?

Urinary symptoms are the most common complaints in men with prostate cancer, although early, curable prostate cancer usually produces no symptoms. Most cases originate in the peripheral zone, which is farther away from the urethra than the transitional cell where BPH forms. For this reason, prostate cancer is not as likely to slow down or block urination in its early stages as is BPH (see figure 1–5). When this does occur, however, all of the obstructive symptoms as well as any of the complications of bladder outlet obstruction that were discussed in chapter 5 may occur. In general, *cancer and BPH form in different parts of the prostate.*

The capacity of prostate cancer to metastasize may not be present when the tumor first forms; however, when it does start to spread, the first site appears to be the lymph nodes that surround the prostate.

These peanut-sized lumps are filtering stations that expose materials present in the body's tissue fluids to the immune system. This protective mechanism is able to recognize what is foreign to the body, including cancer cells. The trapping of tumor cells in lymph nodes is a sign that our protective mechanisms are reacting to the prostate cancer cells that have become malignant enough to spread.

Cancer in lymph nodes cannot be felt, but if the nodes become very enlarged, they may squeeze the ureter and prevent urine from leaving the kidney. This blockage of the kidney can lead to *hydronephrosis,* or dilation of the kidney, and even to kidney failure,

FIGURE 6-4
Lymph Nodes Around Prostate

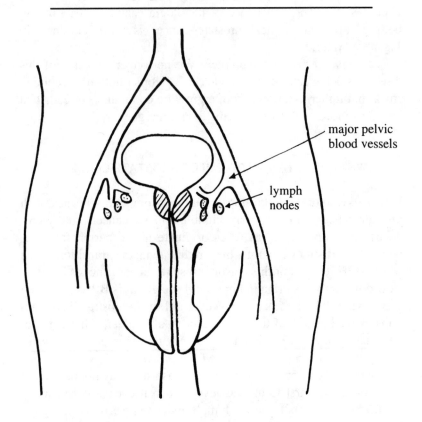

major pelvic
blood vessels

lymph
nodes

which may reveal itself by weakness, vomiting, or other systemic symptoms. Ureteral blockage, which can also occur when prostate cancer grows out of the prostate and directly surrounds the lower ends of the ureters, is the exception in prostate cancer rather than the rule. Although the rectum is also immediately adjacent to the prostate, rectal blockage or injury from direct invasion by prostate cancer is extremely rare. Some patients with dramatic prostate enlargement due to cancer may experience constipation, but this is caused only by the pressure of the prostate mass pushing on the rectum.

When prostate cancers have developed the capacity to metastasize, they do not appear everywhere in the body but show a special predisposition for bone. Research suggests that special growth factors are found in bone that make this location favorable for prostate cancer cells. In patients where spread to the bones has taken place, pain in the pelvis, back, or leg caused by tumors in the bone may be the first symptom of prostate cancer (see figure 2–5).

THE DIAGNOSIS OF PROSTATE CANCER

To the ancient Greeks, diagnosis represented knowledge of a disease through its symptoms—knowledge that was obtained without taking pieces of the patient to the lab. Nowadays, we must insist on information obtained more directly from patients to establish the diagnosis of prostate cancer. Although there are several examinations, blood tests, and X-rays that can point to this disease, they cannot by themselves establish a diagnosis. A prostate biopsy, or removal of a small fragment of prostate tissue, is required.

Prostate Ultrasound and Biopsy

Before transrectal ultrasound came into use, urologists had to feel a nodule in the prostate in order to obtain a biopsy specimen. While this lump was being felt with the finger of one hand, the other hand was used to pass a thin biopsy needle into the suspected nodule after the patient had received some type of anesthetic. Biopsy needles that remove a small sliver of tissue are still used, but we need not rely solely on the sense of touch for guidance.

Transrectal ultrasound, described in chapter 2, passes sound waves at a frequency of about seven thousand cycles per second into the prostate to create a picture in various cross-sections. In about 75 percent of men with cancer, tumors appear as *hypoechoic,* or dark, spots (see figure 3–6). The other 25 percent of men have tumors that blend in with the surrounding tissue and are detected by their effects in distorting the normal prostate architecture. Current technology permits the biopsy needle to be guided into the suspected areas that are seen by ultrasound. This usually requires passing the needle through the wall of the rectum. An automatic device that moves the needle in and out very quickly is used. As the nerve fibers in the rectal wall are sensitive to stretching but not to sharpness, the sensation from the biopsy is minor.

Biopsies performed through the rectum carry the risk of infection, but with antibiotic use, the incidence of significant infection is well below 1 percent. Bleeding in either the bladder or the rectum can occur temporarily after biopsy. While pink urine or bloody spots on toilet paper are fairly common after biopsy, serious bleeding requiring hospitalization is extremely rare. The procedure should not be used with patients who are taking aspirin or other blood thinners. Biopsy needles are not reusable, so there is no risk of contracting a communicable disease from them.

Biopsy needles core out a small sliver of tissue about 15 millimeters (⅝ inch) long. Examination by a pathologist can show how much cancer each core contains. Research has shown that cancers greater than ½ cubic centimeter in volume represent a likely threat of clinical illness. Depending on a patient's age, cancers much smaller than this may represent the "histologic cancer" that is present so frequently in elderly men.

Careful study of the microscopic appearance of these biopsy specimens enables pathologists to give us more information about tumor behavior. There is a system for interpreting the appearance of cancer within the prostate that compares the microscopic architecture of the cancer to that of normal prostate tissue. A scale is used to assign a number from one (looks like normal prostate) to five (bears almost no resemblance to normal prostate) for each area examined. This number is called the *grade* of the cancer and is an indication of how malignant the microscopic appearance of the cells is. Tumor grade ranges from one (*well differentiated:* tumors expected to be slow growing) to five (*poorly differentiated:* tumors at high risk of spreading).

In the commonly used *Gleason System* for grading prostate cancers, the variability of prostate cancer from one area to another is recognized. The grade number from a spot thought to be the most prominent pattern is added to the grade number from a spot repre-

FIGURE 6-5
Tumor Grading

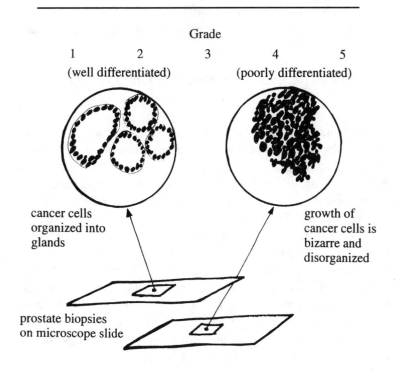

Grade

1 2 3 4 5
(well differentiated) (poorly differentiated)

cancer cells
organized into
glands

growth of
cancer cells is
bizarre and
disorganized

prostate biopsies
on microscope slide

senting the secondary pattern. This results in an overall tumor grade that can range from two (1+1, well differentiated) to ten (5+5, poorly differentiated).

In addition to grade, pathologists now have a tool that affords a new look at the genetic makeup of a tumor. This is measurement of the amount of DNA per tumor cell by use of a technique called *DNA flow cytometry*. Normal cells have two copies of each chromosome and are said to be *diploid* in their DNA content. When DNA is stained with special fluorescent dyes and the cell response to laser light is analyzed, the DNA content of cells can be measured. This allows them to be grouped into tumors with diploid DNA (a normal amount of DNA per cell) or tumors with *aneuploid* DNA (tumors with abnormal amounts of DNA per cell).

Although this information is not part of conventional tumor grade assignment, research is showing that DNA content, or *ploidy*, correlates with prognosis. Patients with diploid tumors appear to have a lower rate of progression or recurrence after therapy than patients with aneuploid tumors.

Can There Be Differences of Opinion Among Pathologists?

By examining the biopsy specimen under a microscope, a *pathologist*—a physician specially trained to recognize abnormal tissues—can make the diagnosis of prostate cancer. The pathologist can use the word "cancer" only when the microscopic appearance of the biopsy tissue meets a set of standard criteria, ranging from the appearance of a single cell to the overall tissue architecture.

In the majority of cases, the microscopic features necessary for the diagnosis of prostate cancer are obvious to the trained observer. Fortunately, diagnosing cancer on a biopsy specimen cannot be an arbitrary individual decision. The determination rests on a series of well-established microscopic features and is reinforced by tissue and cancer committees in hospitals. These groups of doctors, which are a mandatory requirement for hospital accreditation, review and monitor cases involving the diagnosis of the disease.

Infrequently, when the microscopic appearance of a cancer is very unusual, pathologists may request a second opinion by another pathologist who is especially qualified or experienced in urologic diseases. While a second opinion on the treatment of prostate cancer may benefit the patient, obtaining a second opinion on the biopsy interpretation is generally not necessary.

Who Should Undergo Prostate Biopsy?

Biopsy of the prostate should be done in the following cases: (1) the patient is suspected of having prostate cancer, and (2) establishing the diagnosis would influence the patient's subsequent decisions and medical care. The second factor is important in elderly patients with apparently limited disease. As we will discuss, "watchful waiting" or no therapy at all may be appropriate action for a selected group of patients. For such patients, even the suspicion of localized prostate cancer may not warrant biopsy if no specific treatment would be recommended anyway.

Who Is Suspected of Having Prostate Cancer?

For many years, the digital rectal exam was the only means available to check for prostate cancer. If the prostate had an uneven contour, hard spots, or lumps, prostate cancer was suspected. To this time-tested and reliable finding we have now added a blood test: the serum prostate-specific antigen.

PSA

Prostate-specific antigen is the name given to a particular protein secreted in high concentrations by the cells of prostate glands into semen, where it affects seminal viscosity. Very little leaks into the bloodstream, giving normal men a PSA value of less than 4 nanograms per milliliter of blood (1 nanogram = 1 billionth of a gram). When cancer disrupts the architecture of the prostate glandular chambers, more PSA can leak into the bloodstream, causing levels to rise.

This protein is made only by the prostate, so it is prostate-specific. Unfortunately, it is not cancer-specific; an abnormal value does not prove cancer is present. PSA can be elevated with BPH, infection, or inflammation of the prostate, as well.

Higher levels of PSA do increase the likelihood that cancer is present, however. In a group of men with a normal-feeling prostate, 2.5 percent were found to have cancer when the PSA was less than 4 nanograms per milliliter, compared with 32 percent who had cancer when the PSA was greater than 10 nanograms per milliliter. Estimates have placed the likelihood of prostate cancer at approximately 75 percent in patients with a PSA greater than 20 nanograms per milliliter. Normal values for PSA depend on the patient's age. (See Table 6–1.)

The PSA test is a very effective way to track the progress of a man known to have prostate cancer. Its numerical value at the time

TABLE 6–1
PSA: Relations to Age and Cancer

PSA level	Age, with normal values					Chance of finding cancer even if exam result is normal
	40	50	60	70	80	2.5% chance of cancer PSA <4.0
4 —	40–49 (<2.5)	50–59 (<3.5)	60–69 (<4.5)	70–79 (<6.5)		Between PSA of 4 and 10, chance is quite different for different age groups (higher chance in younger men)
10 —						32% chance of cancer PSA >10
20 —						75% chance of cancer PSA >20

of diagnosis can add information about the extent of prostate cancer. Studies have shown that with a PSA of 10 nanograms per milliliter or less at the time of diagnosis, the prostate cancer is extremely unlikely to have spread to the bones. With successful curative removal of a cancerous prostate, the PSA level becomes undetectable, as the body's only source of this protein has been removed. Successful radiation and hormonal therapy also are associated with dropping PSA levels.

Change in PSA values over time may add accuracy in the diagnosis of men with elevated PSA levels. One study showed that with a PSA increase of 0.75 nanograms per milliliter per year, or greater, there was over a 90 percent chance of cancer being present. Since PSA elevation can occur with prostate enlargement due to BPH, comparing the PSA level with the prostate size to get a number known as PSA density may help in distinguishing cancer from BPH. With a PSA density greater than 0.15 nanograms per milliliter per cubic centimeter of prostate size, the likelihood of cancer exceeds 80 percent.

High-Risk Groups

Are blood relatives of a prostate cancer patient, or black men, at sufficient risk of prostate cancer to warrant a biopsy without the presence of telltale symptoms? Certainly, these men are in higher-risk groups, but as individuals they would be suspected of harboring cancer only if they had an abnormal result of digital rectal exam or an abnormally high PSA value. Whether certain groups of men should undergo earlier or more frequent rectal exams and PSA tests is a public policy question that must take many other factors into account.

The patient's age influences suspicion of prostate cancer. Although men over eighty are more likely to have prostate cancer, they are not necessarily in need of prostate biopsy. Minimal irregularities noticed during the rectal exam or incidentally discovered PSA elevations may not warrant biopsy in this group, as finding the small cancers so common in elderly men may have little medical importance. On the other hand, minimal irregularity in the prostate or even a borderline PSA level should mandate biopsy in a forty-nine-year-old man, for example.

Indication for Biopsy

When these and other factors are taken into consideration, prostate ultrasound and biopsy are indicated when the prostate exam result is clearly abnormal and/or the PSA is above 10. A PSA level between 4 and 10 nanograms per milliliter is in an acknowledged "gray zone," where additional clinical judgment is required. The options range from periodic follow-up with repeat PSA tests (in older men) to immediate biopsy (in younger men). PSA values in this range must be interpreted in relationship to the rectal exam: Prostate irregularities that can be felt increase the chances of prostate cancer and should influence the decision to perform biopsy. Again, the rectal exam need not disclose abnormalities for cancer to be present. On the other hand, when a prostate does not feel normal, the PSA level need not be elevated for the physician to recognize the need for biopsy. Approximately 5 to 10 percent of cancers are diagnosed in men with normal PSA levels.

What Is Screening?

Screening is neither seeing a free movie nor window repair, but involves passing all men through a process that will pluck out those who have prostate cancer. It refers to large-scale testing of the public in an attempt to discover prostate cancer at an earlier stage.

Because screening involves mass groups of "normal" men, it is more of a public health policy issue than an individual medical decision. As large-scale policy decisions have an impact on medical and economic fronts, there has been some controversy about screening.

If we had absolute proof that early diagnosis of prostate cancer led to a better health outcome for the population at large, screening programs would be the correct approach. Virtually every doctor involved in the care of prostate cancer patients would agree that cure of this disorder is achieved only in patients with an early diagnosis, and that patients who are not diagnosed until symptoms occur have more advanced disease. Despite these clinical observations, numerical data relating the stage of cancer at diagnosis to overall outcome and cost expenditure do not exist. Policymakers need these figures, and until they are available there will be an ongoing debate. The National Cancer Institute has not endorsed mass screening, nor have consensus conferences on this issue in France, Sweden, or Canada.

The American Cancer Society and the American Urologic Association do recommend that every man over fifty have a yearly rectal exam to check for prostate cancer. Although the PSA test does not presently have FDA endorsement as being "effective in the detection of early prostate cancer," physicians who are well informed about this disease recommend the test be done yearly in conjunction with a rectal exam. A recent study has shown that as a group, men whose cancer was diagnosed by PSA testing have earlier disease, and thereby a greater chance of cure, than those who were diagnosed by rectal exam only.

Prostate cancer is usually curable only in men without symptoms. However, the risks and cost of evaluation and biopsy in those patients who turn out not to have cancer constitute additional considerations for policymakers. In making the decision to screen for a large group, one must consider the effects of disease and testing on the overall health of the group. For a given individual, the choice is simpler. You should weigh, with the help of your physician, the risks of testing against the risks of untreated prostate cancer.

OTHER TESTS WHEN PROSTATE CANCER HAS BEEN DIAGNOSED

Bone Scans

This test, described in chapter 3, is the best way to determine whether prostate cancer has spread to the bones. Because of the biology of prostate cancer, bone is by far the most common site of metastatic or disseminated prostate cancer. Bone scans are used routinely when the result of biopsy shows cancer, although recent evidence suggests that PSA levels may be used to establish the need for a bone scan. When the PSA level is less than 10 nanograms per milliliter, the likelihood of metastatic disease being found by bone scan is extremely low. It has been suggested that a bone scan is not necessary in a man with cancer and a PSA level lower than 10 nanograms per milliliter. Although this may be true, patients with prostate cancer are at risk for developing bone metastases in their lifetime. Obtaining a study as a *baseline* to which further tests are compared can facilitate more accurate interpretation of future studies.

CAT Scans and Magnetic Resonance Imaging (MRI)

Both CAT scans and magnetic resonance imaging (MRI) are capable of depicting the pelvic anatomy that surrounds the prostate. They are not detailed enough to show the structure within the prostate,

TABLE 6–2

Tests Used in Men with a Biopsy Result for Prostate Cancer

Test	What is measured	Problems detected	Usefulness/ Risk	Cost
PSA	Amount of specific protein in blood	Likelihood of spread is related to numerical value	(Usually has been done proir to biopsy)	$40
Transrectal ultrasound	Shape and internal structure of prostate	Useful for measuring size of tumor	(Usually done in conjunction with biopsy)	$800
Bone scan	Areas of skeleton showing increased cellular activity	Metastases, or spread to bones	Very useful/No risk. May not be necessary if PSA <10.	$450
IVP	Anatomy of entire urinary tract	Secondary effects of tumor on bladder/kidneys	Useful when there is blood in urine/Slight risk of allergic reaction	$400
Cystoscopy	Anatomy of urethra and bladder	Source of bleeding from urinary tract	Use only when there is blood in urine/May require anesthesia, pain, stricture	$200
CAT scan	Anatomy of abdomen, pelvis, chest	Lymph node enlargement, tumor spread to other organs	Useful in planning radiation therapy/Minimum risk of allergic reaction	$600
MRI scan	Anatomy of abdomen, pelvis, chest	Lymph node enlargement, tumor spread to other organs. May be helpful in detecting tumor spread through prostate capsule	Useful in planning radiation therapy/Can be uncomfortably confining	$1200
DNA flow cytometry	Amount of DNA in tumor cells	Likelihood of agressive tumor behavior	May help in therapy decision in older patients/None	$120

however, which makes them ineffective for accurately determining whether the cancer is contained within the prostate or has spread through the capsule. When prostate tumors are very large, when injury to adjacent structures is suspected, or when a tumor is associated with a very high PSA level, suggesting spread, either of these studies can help to clarify the situation. They are not routinely used before surgery but are commonly used before radiation therapy as an aid for planning the treatment target.

INTEGRATING TEST FINDINGS: Staging

Once prostate cancer has been detected, it is the doctor's job to assemble the results of examinations and tests into a form that is useful for making decisions about treatment options. A system for integrating clinical and laboratory findings into a scale that reflects the anatomic extent of tumor within the body is called tumor *stage*. This is expressed as a category within a spectrum of possibilities. In prostate cancer, it ranges from *stage A* (small tumors found incidentally) to *stage D* (advanced cancer that has spread). Combined with tumor grade (which reflects cellular appearance), stage, the anatomical extent of a tumor, is essential for determining prognosis and mandatory for planning therapy. Several staging systems are now in use.

The *Whitmore-Jewett* classification has been used the longest. Stage A cancer in this system refers to cancer that cannot be felt on rectal examination. This category was devised to accept the 8 to 10 percent of patients who are incidentally discovered to have prostate cancer when they undergo prostate surgery to relieve blockage due to (presumed) benign enlargement. Further subdivision into A1 cancer (only a few microscopic areas of cancer) and A2 cancer (more diffuse involvement) makes clinical sense, as these different situations have different prognoses. Stage B is cancer felt as a lump or nodule localized to the prostate on rectal exam. This also is subdivided into B1 (nodules less than 1.5 centimeters in size involving only one lobe of the prostate) and B2 (nodules greater than 1.5 centimeters, or involving both lobes). When digital rectal examination discloses hardness or a tumor that extends up into the seminal vesicles or outside the normal boundaries of the prostate, this is called stage C. Stage D cancer has spread out of the prostate, to the lymph nodes only in stage D1, or to bones or other organs in stage D2.

Staging accomplished with physical examination, PSA tests, bone

TABLE 6–3
Cancer Staging Systems

Whitmore-Jewett system	TNM system			
Stage	T (tumor)	N (nodes)	M (metastases)	Meaning
A1	T1a	N0	M0	Can't feel tumor on exam (incidentally discovered by TURP). Minimal amount of tumor present. No lymph node or distant metastases.
A2	T1b	N0	M0	Can't feel tumor on exam (incidentally discovered by TURP). Tumor diffusely present. No lymph node or distant metastases.
B1	T2a	N0	M0	Nodule in prostate 1.5cm or smaller. No lymph node or distant metastases.
B2	T2b	N0	M0	Nodule in prostate greater than 1.5 cm or tumor in both lobes. No lymph node or distant metastases.
C	T3	N0	M0	Tumor mass extends beyond prostate capsule. No lymph node or distant metastases.
D1		N1	M0	Lymph nodes contain cancer but no distant metastases.
D2		N1	M1	Metastases present in lymph nodes and bones, or other parts of the body.

Example: After surgery on a B2 nodule (T2b tumor) showed lymph node involvement, it was reclassified T2bN1M0.

scans, CT scans, and MRI scans is called *clinical staging,* as distinguished from staging information obtained at surgery. Surgically removing the lymph nodes, or *surgical staging,* is the most accurate method of determining whether cancer has spread out of the prostate. Clinical staging usually underestimates the extent of disease compared with surgical staging, as a portion of patients with clinically localized cancer (stages A through C) turn out to have lymph nodes invaded by cancer. The incidence ranges from 10 to 20 percent of patients with stage A2 or B cancer to approximately 50 percent of stage C patients. This finding, which reclassifies these patients into stage D1, has a profound influence on prognosis. Eighty percent of patients with lymph node metastases will develop further spread into the bones within four to five years, compared with approximately 20 percent of men who have lymph nodes free of cancer.

In an effort to establish an international standard that gives stage information about the primary tumor (within the prostate), the lymph nodes, and metastatic disease, the *TNM system was devised.* The tumor (T category) is subdivided into T1, T2, or T3 depending on the extent of tumor within the prostate. These are further subdivided into T1a, T1b, T2a, and T2b, as shown in table 6–3. The lymph node (N) category gives the status of the lymph nodes, and the metastases (M) category characterizes the metastatic disease if any is present.

Perhaps the greatest importance of uniform staging is the widespread applicability it lends to the results of clinical trials. When the outcome of therapy or other data on patients with prostate cancer is based on a uniform system of classification, the information from different studies can be combined and compared. This increases understanding and leads to better, more uniform patient care.

Take a Number—But Remain a Person

For the man with prostate cancer, appropriate advice and management can be offered only when all tests have been condensed into two numbers: grade and stage. The cellular form of the tumor and its anatomical extent are key factors in predicting outcome with or without treatment. Despite the utility of these categories, they do not contain sufficient information to enable the determination of medical care. Every person is different, and the statistical predictions that come from observations of groups of patients remain most accurate when used in the same way—on groups of patients. Predicting an individual's future is uncertain, which makes the human context essential for decision making. General health, age, sexual interest, and ability to deal with risk must be used to put tumor grade and stage in a perspective that will produce effective and compassionate medical care.

TREATMENT OF PROSTATE CANCER

What Happens If Prostate Cancer Is Not Treated?

In untreated early prostate cancer, there is usually a slow inexorable growth of the tumor. One study showed that in patients with stage B cancers, the time needed for the tumor to double in size was more than four years. In another study of localized prostate tumors followed up for a ten-year period without treatment, tumor growth within the prostate was the most common observation. In this group of men, all showed enlargement of the prostate tumor, yet only 20 percent developed metastases, and half of them died. A large group of Swedish men with localized cancer was recently studied. After ten years, 13 percent of the two hundred twenty-three patients had died of cancer. About half of the patients in this group showed signs of progression, and most of them received hormone treatment. In this group, men under seventy showed a progression rate of 75 percent. Although the study confirms that local growth is more common than aggressive spread in early prostate cancer, this group of Swedish men was not representative of patients who are generally considered for aggressive local treatment in this country. The men were older (seventy-two years on the average), and there was a higher proportion of low-grade cancers. A third of the patients had A1 disease, and only 4 percent of the cancers were high grade. Another group of one hundred twenty-two men with favorable (low-grade) cancers and low stage (A and B) disease were followed up for ten years without treatment. Sixty-nine percent of these men developed tumor growth out of the prostate (progression to stage C), 28 percent developed metastases, and 16 percent died of prostate cancer.

Over a ten-year period, localized cancers (stages A and B) are more likely to enlarge locally and spread to bones than to kill. Not all men are initially diagnosed with localized disease, however. An American College of Surgeons survey showed that 23 percent of men are initially diagnosed with stage A cancer, 34 percent of men with stage B, 20 percent of men with stage C, and 24 percent with stage D. In keeping with what we know about tumor biology, the larger and more advanced a cancer is, the more rapidly it accumulates the errors of growth control that render it lethal. An early cooperative study from the Veterans' Hospital showed that after twelve years, only 32 percent of men with stage C cancer were still alive, although many died of other causes. In the same time frame, all but 15 percent of men with untreated stage D cancer had died, about half of them from prostate cancer. In another group, the ten-year survival rate in men with untreated stage D1 cancer (lymph node metastases) was 45 percent. In a group of two hundred thirty-one men with untreated D2 cancer (bone metastases), only 6 percent were alive after three years.

Who Should Be Treated?

Any cancer that can be felt, can be seen on ultrasound, or is capable of elevating the PSA level should be considered for treatment in a man whose life expectancy exceeds ten years. Making treatment decisions about prostate cancer is complicated by the wide range of possibilities this disease can produce. As a doctor, when I care for even one man who is dying of prostate cancer in his early sixties, I want to check every man and aggressively treat every case that appears. Yet for every man whose lifelong retirement plans are set aside to struggle with a terminal illness, there are four or five men with prostate cancer who will continue to go fishing every weekend until something else gives out.

With microscopic prostate cancer so prevalent in older men, there is concern that treating all cases of prostate cancer not only would do more harm than good but would cost us a fortune as well. This concern has been expressed as an opposition to screening all men with PSA tests, which might turn up cancers that otherwise would never be found. These hidden microscopic "histologic" cancers may be well left undiscovered, but tumors that are large enough to be felt, or to be seen on an ultrasound and then subjected to biopsy, are a different story.

Histologic cancers are not different from clinical cancers; they are just smaller. The microscopic cancer found so commonly at autopsy is the same cancer that can lead to illness in a younger man. It is just the later appearance of a disorder that occurs progressively more often as we age. Whenever prostate cancer appears, it displays a slow but relentless growth, which requires a number of years to develop enough cellular anarchy to kill. It has been estimated that

FIGURE 6-6
The Natural History of Prostate Cancer

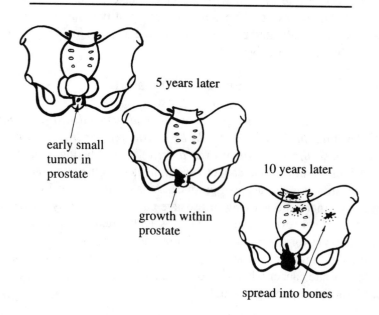

5 years later

early small
tumor in
prostate

10 years later

growth within
prostate

spread into bones

prostate cancer will expand into a larger but still localized tumor over five years, spread or metastasize after eight to ten years, and cause death in twelve to fifteen years. When cancer begins in an elderly man, there simply may not be enough time left in his life span for these events to occur.

From this perspective, and other convincing data as well, it appears that size has an important relationship to the threat of disease progression. Cancers that are less than ½ cubic centimeter in volume are probably at the very beginning of this twelve- to fifteen-year process. In men with a life expectancy less than this, there may be no reason to offer treatment. Tumors smaller than that are difficult to discover with any examination short of an autopsy, however.

Localized Versus Systemic Cancer

Clinical experience and basic science have shown that prostate cancer can exist in two different forms: localized cancer and systemic cancer. Although the passage of sufficient time will allow a localized cancer to progress and spread, there is good evidence that effective treatment of a localized tumor before this occurs can result in cure. For this reason, selecting treatment options depends on the extent, or stage, of the cancer.

TREATING LOCALIZED CANCER

The goal in treating localized cancer is complete elimination of the disease when possible. Surgical removal of all cancerous tissue is one accepted way to do this; killing cancer cells with high-energy radiation is the other. Successful surgical removal requires the cancer be localized in the prostate, whereas radiation can still be employed when cancer has pushed through the capsule and into the seminal vesicles. When malignant cells have left the prostate and spread to the lymph nodes, there is no good evidence that any aggressive local therapy (surgery or radiation therapy) can eliminate the disease from the body.

TABLE 6-4

Treatment Options: Localized Cancer

Rx	Indications	Contraindications	Side effects and complications	Results	Cost
Watchful Waiting	Any man with A1 tumor; any man with less than 10-year life expectancy and A2 or B Tumor	Stage C cancer with symptoms, stage B cancer in men with greater than 10 years life expectancy	Risk of progression: up to 35% of untreated stage B tumors will spread in 5 years	Recent study showed only 13% of older men died of cancer in 10-year observation period	$200/year
Radical Prostatectomy	Stage A2 or B cancers in men with a 10-year life expectancy or greater	Stage C cancers, cancers metastatic to lymph nodes or other sites	Transfusion and anesthesia, impotence, incontinence	15-year survival = 50% (same as men without cancer) in B1 tumor; drops to 25% in B2 tumors	$15,000
Radiation therapy	A2, B, or C cancers	Cancer metastatic to lymph nodes or other sites. Previous pelvic radiation, preexisting colitis or rectal diseases	Rectal irritation or injury, impotence, 50% chance of positive biopsy result 2–3 years after therapy	15-year survival = 28% for all B tumors, 20% for C tumors	$10,000
TURP	Blockage due to cancer when radical prostatectomy is not feasible	Stage B cancer in man with more than 10-year life expectancy	Transfusion, incontinence, stricture, impotence	Does not cure cancer—only improves symptoms due to blockage	$4,000
Hormone therapy	Stage C cancer with short life expectancy (elderly patient)	Curable cancer in patient with life expectancy >5 years	Hot flashes, loss of libido, impotence	Does not cure cancer but will often shrink tumor	$1200
Cryotherapy or Hyperthermia	Localized cancer in patient not candidate for conventional therapy	Unknown	Unknown	Unknown	?

Surgery

Over the years that surgery has been used to treat prostate cancer, many refinements have improved the operation. It is still the most invasive of treatment options and is used more frequently in the United States than in Europe. It is reserved for men who are in reasonably good health and have a life expectancy of at least a decade. Surgical removal of the prostate gland, or radical prostatectomy, should be preceded by removal of lymph nodes to determine whether the disease has spread outside the prostate. Most authorities concur that radical prostatectomy as a cure is indicated only if the lymph nodes are not cancerous. Most surgeons check the lymph nodes through the same incision at the time of surgery. A smaller group of surgeons prefer to sample lymph nodes using a *laparoscope,* which enables the abdominal cavity to be inspected without a large incision. If the lymph nodes turn out to be negative for cancer, the patient undergoes surgical removal of the prostate later.

Radical prostatectomy can be done through a lower abdominal incision (*retropubic* route) or through an incision in the perineum. (These procedures are covered more thoroughly in chapter 7.) When the tumor is removed and sent to the pathologist, it is painted with something similar to India ink. This stains all the outer edges, or margins, of the prostate, permitting them to be identified on the subsequent microscope slides. When slides are made of this tissue, it is then possible to determine whether the cancer cells extend beyond this dyed area or are contained entirely within it.

If the cancer has not spread to the margins, the likelihood of cure with surgery is very high. If the margins are involved, the chance of cure drops. Additional postoperative radiation treatment is often recommended when the margins are cancerous. This may prevent recurrence at the site of surgery, although its long-term effect on survival is unknown.

Radiation Therapy

Radiation therapy relies on the capacity of high-energy X-rays to kill cancer cells. This form of treatment is usually delivered by an

Figure 6-7
Margins in Cancer Removal Surgery

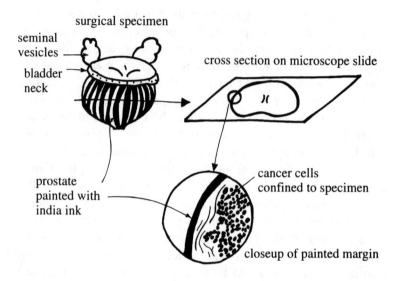

surgical specimen

seminal vesicles

bladder neck

cross section on microscope slide

prostate painted with india ink

cancer cells confined to specimen

closeup of painted margin

external beam of radiation, traveling from a source in a linear accelerator to the patient through controlled access areas, or *ports,* on the patient's body. By careful placement of these ports and limitation of beam size, radiation effect on normal tissues is minimized. The injurious effects of radiation on noncancerous tissue are related to the cumulative dose of radiation received. When radiation beams are sent through different parts of the body and converged on the prostate, the amount of radiation to the cancer is maximized and the amount affecting the surrounding normal anatomy is kept to a minimum. Treatment is given in daily small amounts, or *fractions,* spaced over six or seven weeks. This allows *tumoricidal* (cancer-killing) amounts of radiation to accumulate in the prostate without seriously damaging the skin or surrounding organs.

Selective radiation of the prostate has also been accomplished by implanting radioactive particles into the prostate. The substances currently used for this approach are iodine 125 and palladium 103. Radiation treatment by implant has the theoretical advantage of delivering higher doses to the prostate than could be safely given by external beam methods. The amount of radiation given to the prostate by implants can be three times the amount that external beam methods would permit. Early enthusiasm for this technique waned, however, as results failed to show a clear advantage. Some radiation therapists believe that earlier implant methods did not distribute the particles evenly enough throughout the prostate, and are now studying the use of ultrasound and other techniques to improve the distribution pattern of implants within the prostate.

Radiation is often recommended for men with localized cancer and a life expectancy of ten years or more who have medical problems that would increase the risk of surgery. In addition, radiation is

FIGURE 6-8
Radiation Therapy

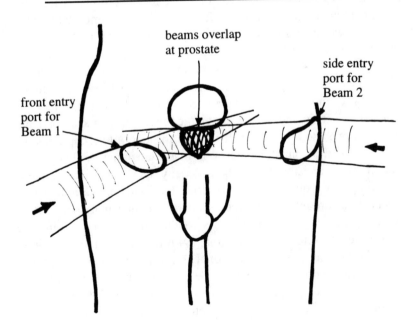

used more frequently than surgery in patients who have locally advanced cancer or stage C disease.

The risks of radiation therapy include a variety of rectal problems, ranging from mild diarrhea to rectal injury with stricture and chronic bleeding. Fortunately, these are not common. Other risks include bladder irritation with chronic frequency or bleeding, and intestinal obstruction. Radiation therapy may be associated with the risk of disease persistence, although the practical implications of this are not known. Some studies have shown that 50 percent or more of men treated with radiation therapy will still have positive biopsy results for cancer two to three years after treatment. This runs parallel to the 40 percent of men who have undergone surgery for prostate cancer and show spread outside the prostate capsule. Both these conditions are thought to increase the chances of subsequent cancer recurrence.

Like surgery, radiation therapy is ineffective for the treatment of prostate cancer that has spread to the lymph nodes. Surgical removal of lymph nodes, or *lymphadenectomy,* is not usually performed on patients who have chosen radiation, as it adds additional risk to the treatment plan. The information it provides may be important, however. As we have discussed, the incidence of lymph node involvement ranges from 20 to 50 percent in stage B2 and C cancers. Lymph nodes are more likely to be involved in patients with high Gleason grades, high PSA values, or aneuploid DNA. In patients with these findings, a staging procedure prior to radiation therapy should be considered. Laparoscopic node sampling in such patients is becoming more common. It is done through a telescopic instrument by use of puncture incisions in the abdomen, rather than a larger single incision. It may be less risky than open surgery, and it certainly has a quicker recovery time. Its disadvantage is that it is conducted through the *peritoneal cavity,* or intestinal space. Standard surgical lymphadenectomy is conducted without exposing the intestinal space to surgical trauma. With a laparoscopic procedure, there is a higher chance of intestinal complications such as injury or postoperative bowel obstruction due to adhesions. It is important to emphasize that a staging operation, be it open surgical lymphadenectomy or laparoscopic lymphadenectomy, is a diagnostic procedure only and has no therapeutic value.

Watchful Waiting

Because of the prolonged growth pattern of prostate cancer, patients with early or localized disease and short life expectancy may reasonably decline aggressive local treatment (surgery or radiation). This does not mean their condition should be ignored, however. Patients choosing this option should be monitored with examination and PSA tests at intervals, for progression to a more advanced stage may warrant other types of therapy. Choosing "watchful waiting" is basically a gamble that aging will produce a cause of death other than prostate cancer. This may be a safe bet and a wise choice in certain cases, but it should be elected only after consideration of all the possibilities.

With a localized cancer, the main criterion for choosing observation rather than surgery or radiation is life expectancy. Over a ten-year span, a man in his sixties with early prostate cancer stands a 50 to 60 percent chance of dying of cancer. Advancing age increases the chances of dying of some other cause, diminishing the statistical threat that prostate cancer will be the cause of death. The decision to forgo aggressive treatment must weigh more than competing causes of death, however. The resulting quality of life must also be taken into account: effects of treatment (such as impotence), the illness and pain that disease progression can cause, and the side effects of treatments that would be mandatory if symptomatic metastases occur. Observation alone is not an option for painful metastases. "Watchful waiting" is not really a "no therapy" option; it is trading early therapy for the possibility of delayed therapy for metastases, if the patient lives long enough. When life expectancy is less than ten years, this choice may be reasonable. In addition, for "watchful waiting" to be chosen, anxiety over possible risks of surgery or radiation must outweigh the anxiety of living with untreated cancer.

One recent study used computer modeling to compare the life expectancies of men treated with aggressive local therapy to "watchful waiting"—observation until the disease spread, then treatment for metastatic disease. An attempt was then made to adjust those figures for quality of life. This paper was not a compilation of clinical observations; it was a computer-generated decision analysis based on several theoretical assumptions. The computer predicted that for the groups as a whole (including older men), aggressive local therapy added only about a year to life expectancy. For younger patients with higher grades of cancer, however, as many as four additional years of life expectancy were predicted. This study was helpful in showing that while men in their sixties benefit from aggressive local therapy, surgery and radiation have little to offer the patient who is older than seventy-five. Whether the years added by treatment are of lesser quality should be for patients, not computers, to decide.

Experimental Therapy

There are new approaches to the control of localized prostate cancer, such as freezing the prostate, or *cryotherapy*. Because of the slow and relentless natural history of prostate cancer, the results of treatment have meaning only when measured ten years or more afterwards. For this reason, there is at present no evidence that these new treatments are truly effective. Until reliable scientific data have been gathered, cryotherapy and other new techniques should be considered experimental.

TREATMENT OPTIONS WHEN CANCER HAS SPREAD

Cancer cells that have lost most regulatory controls are beyond the point of simply growing a gradually enlarging tumor within the prostate. Fortunately, these highly malignant cancer cells can still be affected by treatment. Therapy for advanced prostate cancer that is no longer localized must alter the conditions for tumor growth throughout the body.

Hormone Deprivation

Research in the 1930s and 1940s showed that like normal prostate cells, prostate cancer growth is usually affected by the levels of the male sex hormone testosterone. The Nobel Prize for medicine was awarded to Dr. Charles Huggins in 1966 for demonstrating, in collaboration with Clarence Hodges in 1941, that *orchiectomy,* or removal of both testes, could dramatically improve the condition of men with metastatic prostate cancer. Although we have newer methods of changing the body's hormone environment, the only truly effective therapy for metastatic prostate cancer continues to use the principles discovered by Huggins and Hodges.

Orchiectomy

Removal of both testes is a short (twenty-minute) operation that can be performed as an outpatient procedure. Compared with lifelong use of hormone-suppressing drugs, it is relatively inexpensive. Some patients find this operation psychologically unacceptable, however. As is true of any therapy that dramatically reduces serum testosterone levels, orchiectomy produces loss of libido and may result in hot flashes, slight weight gain, and impotence. It will not change a man's voice or alter his appearance.

Testosterone is produced by the *Leydig cells* within the testes. They are controlled by a pituitary hormone called *luteinizing hormone* and produce about 90 percent of the body's hormone supply. The other 10 percent is contributed chiefly by the adrenal gland. Orchiectomy dramatically reduces the testosterone level in the bloodstream but does not eliminate it altogether.

Drugs That Stop the Formation of Testosterone

It is now possible to stop the testes from producing testosterone by interfering with the chemical message that the brain sends to the pituitary gland to turn on hormone production. The testicular Leydig cells require a pituitary messenger hormone, luteinizing hormone (LH), in order to make testosterone. The pituitary gland releases LH only under the influence of a brain chemical called LHRF *(luteinizing hormone releasing factor).* Two drugs, *goserelin acetate* and *leuprolide,* affect the pituitary gland's response to this chemical signal, thereby reducing its output of LH. This lowers the serum

TABLE 6-5
Treatment Options When Cancer Has Spread

Rx	Indications	Action	Side effects and complications	Results	Cost
Watchful waiting	Not indicated: Hormone therapy is appropriate for frail and elderly				
Radical prostatectomy	Not indicated				
Radiation therapy	Treatment of painful metastatic sites in bones	Tumor destruction or inhibition	Skin irritation, bone marrow, depression	Good for relieving pain	$2,500
TURP	Blockage of bladder due to tumor in prostate	Opens up urethra	Incontinence, bleeding, stricture, impotence	Good for relieving blockage	$4,000

Hormone therapy

1. Orchiectomy	Metastatic cancer	Reduces blood testosterone level	Hot flashes, loss of libido, impotence	Excellent response: tumor regression in about 85% of patients	$2,000
2. Lupron® or Zoladex®	Metastatic cancer	Reduces blood testosterone level	Hot flashes, loss of libido, impotence	Excellent response: tumor regression in about 85% of patients	$500/monthly
3. Eulexin	Metastatic cancer	Blocks the effect of testosterone on cancer cells	Diarrhea, stomach upset, liver injury	Less impotence, but less effect on cancer	$150/monthly
4. Eulexin® + 1 or 2 above	Metastatic cancer	Reduction and blocking of testosterone	Hot flashes, loss of libido, impotence, diarrhea, stomach upset, liver injury	Prolonged survival compared with 1, 2 or 3 alone	$175–650/ month
Chemotherapy	Metastatic cancer that doesn't respond to hormones	Inhibit or kill cancer cells	Intestinal problems, infections, altered immunity, bone marrow, depression	Poor: Less than 25% response rate	$200/month
Cryotherapy or hyperthermia	Blockage due to primary tumor in prostate	Tumor destruction	Rectal injury, treatment failure	Not as good or predictable as TURP	Unknown

testosterone to the same low levels that are obtained after orchiectomy. Both of these drugs can produce loss of libido, impotence, and hot flashes. Less commonly, they produce other side effects such as diarrhea, indigestion, headache, or breast tenderness. They are given as a monthly injection on a lifelong basis.

Estrogen Therapy

Before the introduction of goserelin acetate and leuprolide, *diethylstilbestrol* (DES) was in common use as an alternative to orchiectomy for men with metastatic prostate cancer. This "female hormone" interferes with normal pituitary gland function, reducing testosterone to the same low levels obtained with orchiectomy. In addition to hot flashes and loss of libido, it can produce breast enlargement and a dangerous tendency toward abnormal blood clotting, resulting in heart disease and blood clots in the legs and lungs. For this reason it is seldom used anymore.

Drugs That Block the Effects of Testosterone

Knowing that 10 percent of the body's testosterone output continues after orchiectomy or the administration of leuprolide (or goserelin acetate), researchers have investigated how this small remaining stimulus to cancer growth could be stopped. There are two drugs, flutamide and cyproterone acetate, that act peripherally on prostate cancer cells, blocking the effect of testosterone at the cellular level. This should be distinguished from the other drugs we have discussed that act on the central control of hormone production and lessen the amount of hormone present in the entire body. Flutamide (Eulexin®, Schering) is FDA-approved for use in the treatment of prostate cancer, and most clinical experience in the United States has been with this drug. It is generally employed in combination with orchiectomy, leuprolide, or goserelin acetate. Some patients develop diarrhea or evidence of liver injury while receiving this medication, but this is uncommon. Cyproterone acetate is more widely prescribed in Europe and Canada and is also relatively well tolerated.

Drugs That Affect the Production of Testosterone From the Adrenal Gland

Studies are under way that examine the effects of removing the last 10 percent of testosterone remaining in the bloodstream after orchiectomy or drug therapy. For this to be done, the adrenal production of testosterone must be stopped. Two drugs, aminoglutethimide and ketoconazole, effectively block adrenal testosterone production. These drugs have substantial toxicity, and their overall use remains to be determined.

Chemotherapy

Drugs that interfere with cancer cell growth or metabolism in a nonhormonal way are generally not effective against prostate cancer. Since the prognosis is not good in those patients who have tumor progression despite hormone deprivation, chemotherapy has been used in some of them. However, the results of this strategy have not been encouraging.

TREATMENT RESULTS AND RECOMMENDATIONS

Stage A

About 10 percent of men who undergo prostate removal for blockage caused by apparent benign enlargement are found to have cancer in the tissue removed. Patients with stage A cancer have a normal digital rectal exam—no lumps or nodules can be felt. When cancer is present diffusely through the tissue removed at surgery, or is of high Gleason grade, this is called stage A2. When moderate or low-grade cancer (Gleason grade six or less) is found in less than 5 percent of the tissue removed, it is called stage A1 cancer. We now

TABLE 6–6
Treatment Options by Stage

Rx	A1	A2	B1	B2	C	D1	D2
Watchful waiting	Best choice	Reasonable choice in older man with life expectancy less than 10 years; Poor choice in younger men			Only in elderly men without symptoms	Poor choice	
Radical prostatectomy	Usually not necessary	Best choice for healthy men <70 years old; Reasonable choice for men with >10-year life expectancy		Good choice healthy men <70 years		Not indicated	
Radiation therapy	Usually not necessary	Reasonable choice for healthy men <70 years; Best choice for men with life expectancy less than 10 years			Good choice	Good choice for treating metastatic tumors causing pain, not indicated for treating prostate	
TURP	(TURP has already been done to make diagnosis of A1 or A2 cancer)		Fair choice in patient who has chosen watchful waiting and develops symptoms of blockage		Good choice for blockage of bladder due to tumor (TURP can relieve blockage but not cure cancer)		
Hormone therapy		Usually not applicable			Good choice in elderly patient		Best choice

have a third group of patients with prostate cancer and a normal result of digital rectal exam—those who are diagnosed by ultrasound-guided biopsy when the PSA level is found to be elevated. Although there is no established category for this in conventional staging systems, some have called this stage A3 prostate cancer.

Most studies have shown that men with stage A1 prostate cancer have a life expectancy very similar to that of men of the same age without prostate cancer. In one study of over one hundred men, only 10 percent had conditions that progressed over a prolonged follow-up, and cancer claimed the lives of only 1 percent of these men. Clearly, in this case, disease progression does not mean death. The majority of patients with stage A1 cancer require no therapy. They should be monitored with periodic rectal exams and PSA levels and perhaps studied with ultrasound if these reveal changes over time. Patients with A1 cancer who are under sixty should be followed up more closely. Some feel that in limited circumstances, these men may be candidates for radiation therapy or radical surgery, although studies have shown that aggressive therapy benefits only a small minority of men with stage A1 cancer.

In contrast to the favorable outlook for stage A1 cancer, men with stage A2 cancer are at substantial risk for disease progression or cancer-related illness and death. Approximately 20 to 30 percent of men with stage A2 cancer have lymph node metastases at the time of diagnosis. Theirs is a higher-volume, more aggressive form of prostate cancer. For this reason, any patient with stage A2 cancer and a life expectancy of ten years or more is a candidate for radiation or surgery. If he is proved to have lymph node metastases during the course of staging evaluation or surgery, he is reclassified as stage D1 prostate cancer.

Patients whose prostate feels normal but are found to have cancer based on a high PSA level are probably in a similar group to those with stage A2 cancer. Although clinical experience with PSA levels as a staging tool is still being gathered, evidence suggests that these patients should be considered for radical prostatectomy or definitive radiation therapy when their life expectancy is ten years or more.

Stage B

In patients with these cancers, a small lump is felt in the prostate, but staging tests show no evidence of spread. Nodules that are confined to one-half of the prostate and are smaller than 1.5 centimeter are termed stage B1 cancers. When a nodule involves both lobes of the prostate or is greater than 1.5 centimeter in size, it is called stage B2. Both of these categories have tumors that are confined to the prostate without identifiable extension into adjacent structures such as the seminal vesicles. In general, stage B prostate cancer has a likelihood of progression and cancer-related death if untreated for too long. When life expectancy exceeds ten years, aggressive local therapy is warranted.

Ten to 15 percent of stage B1 patients and 20 to 30 percent of stage B2 patients have lymph node metastases at the time of surgery. In general, neither radical prostatectomy nor radiation is curative in men with lymph node involvement.

Patients with stage B1 disease and more than ten years' life expectancy have a greater probability of disease-free survival with radical prostatectomy than with radiation. The fifteen-year tumor-free survival rate for patients with stage B1 cancer is 50 percent with radical prostatectomy, which slightly exceeds the results obtained with radiation therapy and nearly matches the expected fifteen-year survival rate of healthy men in this age group. By comparison, approximately 35 percent of untreated stage B1 patients will develop metastases within five years.

The fifteen-year tumor-free survival rate for patients treated surgically for stage B2 cancer is about 25 percent, which is similar to the results obtained with radiation. As tumor volume increases, so does the chance that at the time of surgery, cancer will have escaped through the capsule or extended out to the margins of surgical resection. This finding, present in up to 40 percent of patients with high-volume, high-grade, clinically localized prostate cancer, increases the risk of eventual recurrence. If we could accurately detect capsular penetration by some type of testing, it would be wise to reserve surgery only for patients with cancer that is still within the capsule. Since there are no accurate tests for this, and since cancers with minimal capsular extension may still be curable by surgery, the decision for surgery versus radiation therapy in stage B2 cancers is largely one of individual choice. The one comparative study of surgery versus radiation for stage B cancer showed slightly better results with surgery, although some investigators feel there were shortcomings that weakened the conclusions of the study. To paraphrase one authority, the optimal management of clinically localized prostate cancer is still more a matter of opinion than of fact. A study of nationwide trends has shown that radical prostatectomy is being used more often for localized prostate cancer. Because of technical improvements in this procedure, it can now be conducted with quite a low risk, and it offers the best chance of cure if the tumor turns out to be truly confined to the prostate.

Stage C

This category encompasses tumors that have spread outside the prostate capsule, usually into the seminal vesicles. Patients who have undergone radical prostatectomy for what appeared to be stage B disease, and are found by the pathologist's examination of removed tissues to have cancer extending into the seminal vesicles or outside the prostate capsule, are reclassified to this group. These patients are said to have *surgical stage C* cancer, in comparison with those who, on clinical examination only, had evidence of tumor extension, or *clinical stage C* cancer. When surgery has been done, about 50 percent of patients with clinical stage C cancer will turn out to have lymph node metastases, which would reclassify them to *surgical stage D1* disease.

There is some evidence that postoperative radiation therapy in patients with surgical stage C cancer may lessen the chance that the cancer will recur, although this is controversial. In general, patients with clinical stage C cancer cannot be cured by radical surgery even if the lymph nodes turn out not to be cancerous. For this reason, radiation has often been recommended as the treatment of choice for clinical stage C patients. The results of radiation have ranged from a 64 percent five-year survival rate to a 20 percent fifteen-year survival rate. However, when the time to the first development of metastases was measured in a group of stage C patients treated with radiation, it was found to be the same as in a group of men who received no therapy. This has led some investigators to question the utility of radiation therapy in patients with locally extensive prostate cancer.

Patients with clinical stage C cancer commonly develop urinary obstruction due to compression of the urethra by the bulky tumor. A transurethral resection of the prostate (TURP), or surgical resection of the prostate via the urethra, may be performed. It is effective in relieving this obstruction, but if radiation therapy has already been given, TURP represents a 30 percent risk of urinary incontinence. Because of this, many urologists feel that a TURP followed by some form of hormonal deprivation (see below) is optimal therapy for patients with stage C cancer who have symptoms of bladder obstruction.

Stage D

Cancer involving the lymph nodes, without evidence of further spread, is termed stage D1. Although the cancer still seems to be anatomically localized (to those lymph nodes in the pelvis), the lymph node involvement in fact represents the first evidence that tumor growth has spread out of the prostate and become a system-wide problem. We know this because despite any type of aggressive local therapy (radiation or surgery), patients with D1 cancer will eventually develop distant metastases, or stage D2 cancer.

If testosterone levels in the bloodstream are reduced and the effect of testosterone on cancer cells is blocked, the growth of prostate cancer anywhere in the body can be slowed. Unfortunately, this is not a cure, since prostate cancer can eventually produce a group of cancer cells that no longer require hormonal support for growth. This leads to the much more serious condition of *hormonally unresponsive prostate cancer,* which cannot be effectively treated by any known means. On the average, the emergence of this unresponsive form of cancer takes two to three years to develop from the time hormonal therapy is begun. There is a considerable range, however, based in part on how much cancer is present at the time therapy is started. While one third of patients with hormonally treated metastatic cancer will develop progression within the first twelve months because of the emergence of hormonally resistant disease, 5 to 15 percent of men with hormonally treated metastatic prostate cancer live ten years or longer.

The cornerstone of hormonal therapy for metastatic prostate cancer is reduction of the blood level of testosterone by 90 to 95 percent. This can be accomplished by orchiectomy, monthly injections of leuprolide or goserelin acetate, or the daily administration of DES pills. The result of any of these methods on hormone levels is equivalent, but the rapid reduction in hormone levels achieved with orchiectomy makes it preferable in certain situations. It is recommended in patients with metastatic prostate cancer when tumor deposits in the spine threaten to compress and injure the spinal cord, or when tumor bulk in the pelvis obstructs the ureters and causes kidney impairment. Orchiectomy will eliminate 90 to 95 percent of testosterone from the bloodstream in three hours, providing a rapid effect on metastatic tumors. Leuprolide and goserelin acetate both affect the pituitary gland to cause a transient increase in blood testosterone levels, which can temporarily worsen the situation. Although this effect can be blocked by the use of flutamide, the overall effect is slower than that of orchiectomy. Any of these methods of dramatically reducing circulating testosterone levels will produce *remission* or objective improvement in 80 percent of men with stage D2 prostate cancer.

Because the remission brought about by hormone deprivation in metastatic prostate cancer does not last forever, the use of orchiectomy or medications was formerly delayed until clear-cut symptoms of metastases, such as pain from bone tumors, were present. More recent evidence suggests that delaying hormone therapy is not a good idea. Survival may be prolonged in patients with stage D cancer by starting hormonal therapy at the time the metastases are diagnosed rather than waiting for symptoms to appear. There is little question that immediate hormone therapy is indicated for anyone with stage D2 cancer.

The hormonal management of patients with stage D1 cancer is more controversial. Although 80 percent of these patients will progress to stage D2 within five years, we do not have irrefutable evidence that starting hormonal therapy when the lymph node cancer is diagnosed will prolong life more than if hormonal therapy is started when progression to stage D2 occurs. Indirect evidence favors the early start of hormonal therapy. It appears that hormone therapy begun when the lymph nodes are diagnosed may have an advantage, but we have to consider quality-of-life issues as well. Cancer in the lymph nodes will not affect the potency of a sexually active man, but hormonal deprivation will reduce libido, probably will cause impotence, and may reduce the overall energy level. Because of this, a sexually active man with stage D1 cancer may wish to spend the next five years in a more normal functional capacity rather than opting for a possible or theoretical prolongation of life span. For a man with stage D1 cancer who is not sexually active, early hormonal therapy is probably the best option.

The use of *antiandrogen* medication such as flutamide (Eulexin®, Schering) without orchiectomy or other forms of hormone deprivation may be considered in the sexually active man with stage D1 cancer, but caution is necessary. Since these medications block the effect of testosterone on the cancer cell without changing the blood level of testosterone, when used alone they are less likely to cause impotence than orchiectomy or monthly injections of leuprolide or goserelin acetate. Studies have shown that antiandrogens used alone are clearly less effective in controlling mestastatic cancer than orchiectomy or leuprolide or goserelin acetate. Some researchers believe that using these drugs alone, without lowering the serum testosterone level, may lead to earlier development of hormonally unresponsive cancer. For this reason, the use of flutamide alone to control metastatic cancer with less impact on sexual function should be undertaken only after all the potential risks have been considered. On the other hand, when combined with a treatment that lowers testosterone, these drugs are beneficial.

Since orchiectomy and monthly injections of leuprolide or goserelin acetate attack prostate cancer differently than does flutamide, it makes sense to combine the two. A study recently completed at the National Cancer Institute on six hundred men with metastatic prostate cancer has shown that the combination of either orchiectomy or monthly injections of leuprolide or goserelin acetate with flutamide is more effective than either treatment without flutamide. In the group studied, the researchers found an average survival of thirty-five months when flutamide was combined with leuprolide or goserelin acetate, compared with twenty-eight months when monthly injections of those drugs were used without flutamide.

Unfortunately, there is no uniformly effective therapy for patients with hormonally unresponsive prostate cancer, although some new drugs, such as *suramin,* are currently under evaluation. This is an antiparasitic medication that interferes with cellular growth factors. It has produced responses in some patients with advanced prostate cancer, but it is quite toxic and can be used only within the confines of a controlled clinical trial. For pain control in patients with hormonally unresponsive metastatic cancer, radiation therapy to the involved sites can be helpful.

*   *   *

Because of his father's diagnosis, Jack Chambers' son had double the usual risk of prostate cancer. I recommended that a digital examination and PSA test be done annually, beginning at age forty-five.

Naturally, after reviewing his biopsy result, the grade and staging of his cancer, and his treatment options, Jack had a lot of questions. Underlying them all was a desire to know whether early detection of prostate cancer could lead to cure. I think there is strong evidence for this optimistic outlook, and told him so.

He was back to work four weeks after surgery. When I reviewed his follow-up plan, I am not sure he was listening carefully. I think he was relieved to start worrying about his business again and forget about medicine for a while.

Chapter 7

SURGERY

Advances in technology, from high-quality optical and television systems to improved electronic physiologic monitoring, have increased the safety and effectiveness of prostate surgery. However, other treatment advances have paralleled this evolution, producing a wider variety of nonsurgical therapeutic options. As a consequence, surgery has stepped back from its former preeminent position as the urologist's solitary means of treatment. It continues to play a key role in the management of prostate disorders, however, and is safer, more controlled, and more predictable than ever.

There are two reasons to operate on the prostate: (1) to remove it in its entirety for cure when cancer occurs, or (2) to treat complications of benign prostatic enlargement or cancer. The vast majority of these complications are due to obstruction and are corrected by removing only that part of the prostate responsible for the blockage. Rarely, benign enlargement produces troublesome bleeding, which is also cured by removing the involved part.

Selecting the role surgery will play in a given individual depends on the patient's age, medical condition, personal preferences, and acceptance of risk. Knowledge of other treatment options, some of which have been covered in chapters 5 and 6, is also a prerequisite. The procedure descriptions that follow will fill in some of the technical details and provide additional familiarity with what actually takes place in the operating room.

OPEN VERSUS ENDOSCOPIC SURGERY

Open surgery is the traditional variety, wherein an incision allows the surgeon to directly inspect and feel the anatomical structures involved in the disease process. Endoscopic surgery channels the view through an optical system and eliminates the information gained by touching and feeling. When endoscopic surgery is done through natural anatomical openings (as with the TURP, in which the operating scope is passed through the urethral channel), no incisions are used. Endoscopy of the abdominal cavity, called laparoscopy, requires about four small incisions or puncture sites for the introduction of optical and other instruments into the abdomen.

ANESTHESIA FOR PROSTATE SURGERY

A variety of anesthetic techniques can be used with operations for benign and malignant disorders of the prostate. Contemporary anesthesiology often combines several drugs or methods to eliminate the pain and anxiety of a surgical operation. The other essential function of this science is to provide highly sophisticated physiologic monitoring. To ensure the safety of an operation, many of the body's vital functions are continually monitored. It is the task of the surgeon and the anesthesiologist, working together, to ensure that the only changes occurring during surgery are the planned alterations in anatomy and a reduction in the patient's perception of pain.

Spinal anesthesia is the preferred form of anesthesia for a TURP. By introduction of a local anesthetic similar to Novocain around the lower parts of the spinal nerves within the backbone, the sensation of the lower half of the body can be temporarily blocked. Depending on the drugs used, this effect can last from one to several hours. Spinal anesthesia has the added safety of leaving most of the body's protective reflexes and mechanisms in their normal condition. A light sedative is often used with this technique to reduce anxiety.

Epidural anesthesia is similar in that only one region of the body

FIGURE 7-1
Endoscopy

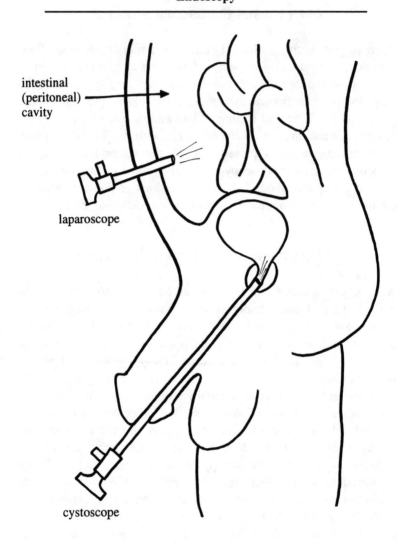

intestinal
(peritoneal)
cavity

laparoscope

cystoscope

is anesthetized. This is accomplished by placement of a tiny tube, or catheter, adjacent to the spinal nerves and the slow introduction of anesthesia or other drugs into this area. In contrast to spinal anesthesia, epidural infusion of pain-killing medication can be continued for several days after surgery. This can produce a completely pain-free recovery. Since pain is usually not a problem after a TURP, epidural anesthesia is used more commonly for open surgical procedures on the prostate.

General anesthesia uses a careful and balanced combination of drugs and gases to induce a nonfeeling, sleeping state. Careful monitoring of several bodily functions allows this state to be regulated according to the needs of the particular operation. Although this method causes more effects throughout the body than regional anesthesia, it also allows closer control of the patient's vital functions.

SURGICAL HARDWARE—DRAINS AND TUBES

Operations for both benign and malignant prostate conditions usually rely on a urinary tube, or catheter, during the healing phase. The catheter may be used from two to three days after a TURP or for three weeks after a radical prostatectomy.

Catheters are made of specially formulated rubber. A Foley catheter is held in place by a balloon that is inflated within the bladder after the tip of the catheter reaches the bladder. This prevents the tube from sliding out.

The balloon has another use following TURP—it can be used to push down on the bladder neck and compress bleeding blood vessels. This is accomplished by mild traction, or pulling on the catheter.

Some catheters have just one channel to allow urine to drain; others have two channels. The second one is used for irrigation, or washing out of the bladder with a constant drip of water. Slow irrigation of the bladder after a TURP allows the blood accumulating within the organ to be diluted and washed out before it can collect and clot, which can block the channel of the catheter and prevent normal drainage of the bladder.

When open surgery is done, such as a radical prostatectomy for cancer, a second type of tube, called a drain, is used. These come in a variety of types but all serve the same purpose. By running out from the site of surgery through a small separate opening in the abdominal wall, they allow blood, urine, or other tissue fluids that leak out and accumulate in the area of surgery to escape.

When the internal area of surgery is kept free of the accumulation of such fluids, faster healing and fewer infections occur. Drains are usually removed five to six days after surgery.

FIGURE 7-2
Foley Catheter

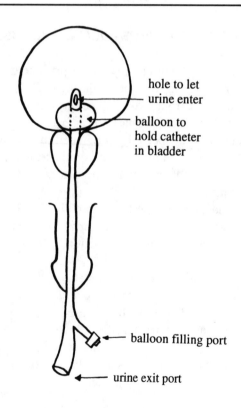

FIGURE 7-3
Surgical Drain

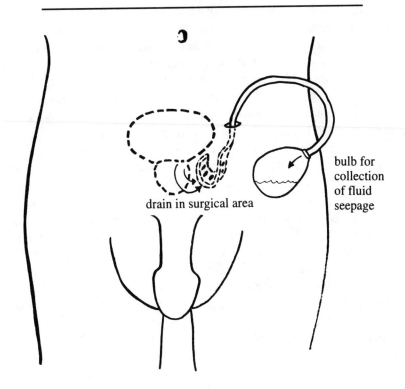

drain in surgical area

bulb for
collection
of fluid
seepage

SURGERY AND TRANSFUSIONS

The need for transfusion during or after surgery depends not only on the amount of blood lost but on the condition of the patient. In general, fewer than one in twenty patients undergoing a TURP require transfusion. In contrast, the average amount of blood lost during a radical prostatectomy is about 1200 milliliters (a little over two pints), and most surgeons end up transfusing these patients.

Although the risk of contacting AIDS, hepatitis, or other diseases from properly screened anonymous donor blood is low, it is prudent to eliminate this risk whenever possible. Since most prostate operations are elective, which means that the patient and doctor both have the luxury of scheduling them at their convenience, most patients can serve as their own blood donors. This process of *autologous blood donation* is fast becoming the standard method in most cases. By donating a pint of blood every week or ten days, a patient can donate three pints of blood in the month prior to surgery. In a relatively healthy patient, the use of iron pills during this period will assist the body in regenerating the blood that has been taken out. The donated blood is carefully labeled and refrigerated until the time of surgery. The maximal amount of time blood can be stored in this way is about forty-five days. After that, it must be frozen. As a rule, the last donation of blood should be more than three days before surgery. Most hospital blood banks will now obtain *directed donor* blood as well, wherein the donors (family members or friends) designate their blood to be held for the use of a specific patient.

To cover the anticipated blood requirement in about 95 percent of cases, one unit (about 300 milliliters) suffices for a TURP, whereas three units are usually advised for a radical prostatectomy. Other than severe anemia or cardiopulmonary disease, the most common reason autologous blood cannot be used for prostate surgery is the preoperative insertion of a catheter. If a man with BPH develops retention and has to have a catheter placed, he may not donate blood as long as the catheter is in. If he is unable to void when the catheter is removed and must wear a catheter until surgery, he will not be able to rely on autologous blood because a catheter can introduce bacteria into the bloodstream. If even a few bacteria are trapped in the donated blood, they have a perfect culture medium to grow in, which causes problems when the blood is transfused back into the patient. This catheter-dependent man with BPH must rely on banked or directed donor blood if he needs it after his TURP, although there is a 95 percent chance he won't.

SURGERY FOR BLOCKAGE

About 90 percent of the surgery done to relieve blockage caused by the prostate is endoscopic, and the vast majority of these cases are for benign enlargement. Prostate cancer can also obstruct the bladder, however. When this occurs in a patient who is not a candidate for removal of the entire prostate for cure, the TURP is an effective means to reduce symptoms due to blockage.

When surgery is done for BPH, only part of the prostate is actually removed: the obstructing inner transitional zone overgrowth. Obstructing tissue is removed in little pieces with a TURP, and in one large piece with open prostatectomy.

TRANSURETHRAL RESECTION OF THE PROSTATE (TURP)

In the United States alone, about four hundred thousand prostatectomies are performed each year. Over 90 percent of these are TURPs, making this the second most common operation performed in the United States. It is most effective in patients with severe symptoms and is particularly successful in restoring urination to those with blockage who are dependent on a catheter. In one study of more than four hundred patients undergoing TURP, symptom improvement was 93 percent in patients with severe symptoms and 79 percent in patients with moderate ones. Compare this to the 30 to 40 percent of patients whose symptoms improved after drug therapy. One of the unexpected results of studying new alternative therapies for BPH has been to remind us just how effective the TURP really is. It is still considered the "gold standard" to which the results of other therapy must be compared. Most studies have shown that surgery results in a doubling (100 percent improvement) in urinary flow rates, compared with about 40 percent improvement resulting from medication. Most urologists would agree that the results with open prostatectomy are at least as good as those obtained with TURP.

Relief of symptoms and improvement in urinary flow seem to last after surgery. One study showed that the flow rates improved by surgery did not decrease in a seven-year follow-up. In time, some patients will experience prostate regrowth and recurrence of symptoms. Statistics show a 13 percent chance of undergoing a second operation if a TURP was done, compared with a 3.5 percent chance if an open prostatectomy was done. This may relate to the difficulty of removing all tissue with an endoscope in patients who have very large prostates and may not reflect the true reoperation rate in most patients undergoing TURP, in whom the size of the gland is more moderate.

Prostate surgery has risks, which has made the recent addition of medicinal therapy for the treatment of BPH most welcome. Certainly, in men with "nuisance" BPH—symptoms but no serious complications—it may be wise to try medication before proceeding with surgery. It is important to recognize how effectively surgery corrects serious complications due to BPH, however. The risks of surgery should not be compared with the risks of medical therapy; they should really be compared with those of unrelieved obstruction, complications of long-term catheter use, infection, and kidney damage that occur in patients for whom surgery is unequivocally indicated. In this analysis, surgery is quite safe. The effectiveness of surgery and its predictability make it a reasonable choice for men with severe symptoms without the complications above and without a prior trial of medication. For these patients, it is not necessary to view surgery as a last resort, to be considered only after medications have failed.

The mortality rate for patients who have had a TURP is about one in one thousand. However, because the procedure is not particularly threatening, candidates for TURP often include elderly men with other medical problems as well. The actual mortality rate for a healthy man in his sixties, for example, is probably much lower.

Recent studies have shown that the risk of succumbing to a heart attack in the ten-year period following surgery is higher for men who have undergone TURP than for those who have undergone open prostatectomy. Although current studies are under way to clarify this finding, many believe that it is also a consequence of patient selection; TURP is safe enough to allow nearly all men with serious blockage to be included (regardless of age or other health problems), while open prostatectomy is usually done only in men healthy enough to undergo this more involved procedure.

The most common complications of prostatectomy are failure of symptoms to improve (10 percent), serious or permanent incontinence (less than 1 percent), infection (10 percent), need for transfusion (5 percent), urethral scarring or stricture (5 percent), loss of erection or impotence (5 to 10 percent), and retrograde ejaculation (90 percent). The last condition is not so much a complication of prostatectomy as an expected consequence. Alteration of bladder neck anatomy by surgery does not stop orgasm or climax, but instead of the semen being expelled down the urethra, it flows back into the bladder (see figure 8–6). This is not harmful, but obviously it can be a problem if a man wants to father children.

Although the TURP originated early in the century, it has kept pace with other technical advances of modern surgery. The optical viewing system is now frequently monitored by high-quality closed-circuit television, which improves the view and saves the urologist's neck. Craning and twisting to peer through a telescope eyepiece during the hour's worth of contortions necessary to perform a TURP has made neck problems an occupational hazard for urologists.

The view through the scope reveals the inner anatomy of the prostatic urethra as it courses from the bladder neck down to the urethral sphincter. Glandular growth is outside the urethra, where it can be detected as a bulging of tissue, pushing inward on the urethra. In lateral lobe hypertrophy, glandular tissue bulges in from either side of the urethra, making the view through this area more like looking through a narrow vertical slot than down a pipe.

Patients often ask how the prostate tissue, which is outside the urethra, can be removed through the urethra. The answer is simple— the urethra is removed along with the tissue. During a TURP, the optical system within the *resectoscope* enables the surgeon to guide a curved loop of wire within the confines of this small space. When the surgeon steps on a pedal, a high-frequency electrical current passes through this wire, which cuts through the tissue. Depending on the shape of the loop and the way it is moved, the result is a "shaving" or chip of tissue being carved out. When the urethra and all the obstructing glandular tissue around it are shaved out, the channel from the bladder neck opens from a narrow ribbon-like slot to a wide passage.

By detecting the change in appearance of the resected tissue, the surgeon can tell how deeply to go in excavating this area, and where the upper and lower limits of resection are. A TURP must remove obstructing tissue from the bladder neck down to a point just above

FIGURE 7-4
**The View of Obstructing Lateral Lobes
Through the Cystoscope**

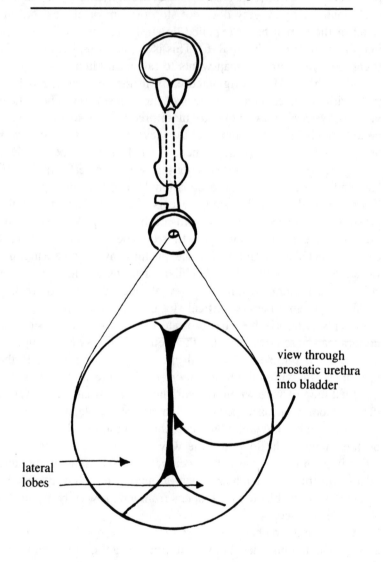

view through
prostatic urethra
into bladder

lateral
lobes

Figure 7-5
TURP (Transurethral Resection of the Prostate)

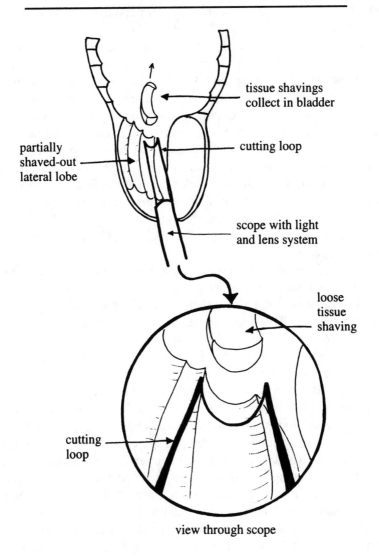

tissue shavings
collect in bladder

cutting loop

partially
shaved-out
lateral lobe

scope with light
and lens system

loose
tissue
shaving

cutting
loop

view through scope

the sphincter. The exit site of the ejaculatory ducts within the prostatic urethra, the *verumontanum,* sits just above the sphincter. If this structure and everything below it are preserved, the sphincter will not be harmed.

At the end of surgery, the channel has opened from the narrow prostatic urethra to the wide prostatic fossa, and the bladder is full of tissue shavings. Using the outer sheath of the resectoscope, with the inner telescope and cutting loop removed, the surgeon can wash out these pieces. The operation is concluded by placement of the Foley catheter, which serves two purposes. It enables the urine to exit without being held up by blood clots in the upper urethra or bladder, and the balloon attached to the catheter may exert gentle pressure down on the bladder neck to stop bleeding in that area. By the time the operation is finished, the surgeon has already stopped most of the bleeding by using a slightly different type of electrical current to the cutting loop, to selectively touch and cauterize any visible bleeding vessels.

Overnight traction downward on the Foley balloon is effective in stopping the ooze from larger veins that are not effectively cauterized in this way. The Foley catheter is usually removed two or three days after a TURP, allowing the patient to return home after a hospitalization that averages three days.

Since most of the prostatic urethra is removed during a TURP, after surgery there is a gap in the membrane that lines the urinary tract. The delicate membrane that covers the inside of the bladder ends at the bladder neck, or upper edge of the resection. Similarly, the membrane lining the urethra channel through the penis ends just above the urinary sphincter. The open space, or *prostatic fossa,* that connects the bladder neck and urethra after TURP is initially a raw area. The bleeding that is normally expected from this area after surgery stops in a day or two as the healing process converts clotted blood into a scab. This crust gradually sloughs off as new lining membrane regenerates to cover the prostatic fossa. Within two to three months, the urinary lining has been regenerated and healing is complete.

Since a TURP removes the overgrown and obstructing transitional zone tissue in small shavings, the length of the operation

FIGURE 7-6
Healing of the Prostatic Fossa

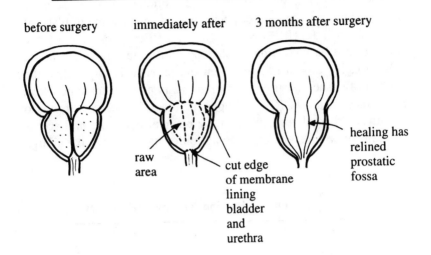

before surgery   immediately after   3 months after surgery

raw area   cut edge of membrane lining bladder and urethra   healing has relined prostatic fossa

varies according to the size of the prostate and the skill of the surgeon. On the average, taking into account the time needed to cauterize blood vessels and irrigate out pieces, he can usually remove about one gram of tissue per minute. The average size of the prostate resected for BPH is about 25 grams, but occasionally it is much larger. If it appears the prostate is so large that a TURP will take more than an hour and a half, another option should be considered. The longer the resectoscope is present in the urethra, the higher is the chance that injury will occur to the urethra and cause a stricture or narrowed area. Also, a prolonged TURP will increase the chance that too much of the irrigating fluid will be absorbed by the body and cause other medical problems.

OPEN PROSTATECTOMY

For obstruction caused by larger amounts of BPH, open prostatectomy is the procedure of choice. It is often called simple prostatectomy to distinguish it from radical prostatectomy, or total removal of the gland. The intent of the open prostatectomy is to relieve obstruction by removing only the transitional zone overgrowth (BPH), leaving the outer peripheral part of the prostate in place. It differs from the TURP by removing the BPH in one solid piece rather than as a collection of shavings. Prostate size is the prime indication for this operation: when the prostate is larger than the amount of tissue the surgeon can remove in an hour to an hour and a half piecemeal (TURP), the open approach is required. It is also employed when abnormalities of the channel make urethral access difficult, or when some other condition of the bladder, like a large

Figure 7-7
Lower Abdominal Incision for Prostate Surgery

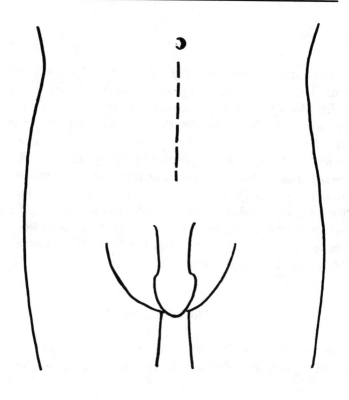

Figure 7-8
Simple Retropubic Prostatectomy

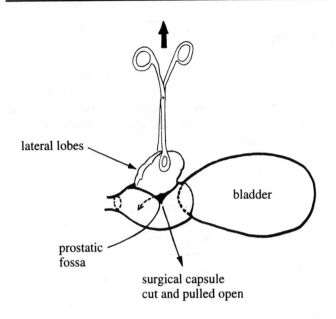

lateral lobes

bladder

prostatic
fossa

surgical capsule
cut and pulled open

bladder stone or diverticulum ("blow out"—see figure 5–10), calls for open surgical repair.

As was discussed earlier, BPH pushes the surrounding prostate tissue outward, stretching it into a shell known as the surgical capsule (see figure 5–3). Open prostatectomy is performed most commonly by one of two approaches: removing the BPH through an incision in the surgical capsule on the front side of the prostate, which lies immediately behind the pubic bone *(retropubic prostatectomy),* or removing the BPH through an incision in the bladder *(suprapubic prostatectomy).* Both operations require a six-inch incision in the lower abdomen, in the area between the pubic bone and the belly button.

When the pelvis is entered for a retropubic prostatectomy, the bladder is seen but not opened up. By pulling it upward and dissecting the fatty tissue behind the pubic bone, the surgeon can see the front of the prostate. An incision in the surface of the prostate that is exposed opens the surgical capsule, allowing the rubbery mass of BPH, including the enclosed prostatic urethra, to be shelled out. This leaves an open space, or prostatic fossa, within the shell of the surgical capsule.

Inspection of this area in the interior of the prostate allows bleeding vessels to be cauterized or oversewn. As is the case following a TURP, the prostatic fossa connects the urethra and the bladder neck. Passing a catheter up the urethra, through the fossa, and into the bladder, followed by sewing the surgical capsule closed, concludes the operation. In addition to the urinary catheter, a drain is placed through a small incision in the abdominal wall to allow any fluids at the site

FIGURE 7-9
**Suprapubic Prostatectomy—The View
Down the "Drain Pipe"**

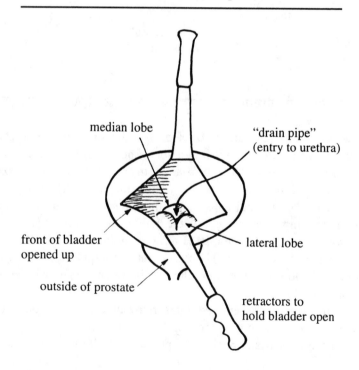

of surgery to exit the patient rather than accumulating inside. Suprapubic prostatectomy is accomplished by making an incision in the wall of the bladder rather than in the prostatic capsule. When the bladder has been opened up, the surgeon can look down "the drain pipe"—the urethra exiting at the bottom of the bladder. This segment of the urethra, together with surrounding encroaching BPH that often bulges up into the bladder, is shelled out of the surgical capsule. After bleeding has been controlled and a catheter placed, the bladder is closed. A drain in the pelvic space is used with this approach as well.

The retropubic approach gives a better view of the prostatic fossa, making control of bleeding vessels a little easier. Because an incision in the bladder muscle is avoided, painful cramping, or *bladder spasm,* are less likely to trouble a patient as he recovers from surgery. The suprapubic approach allows easier removal of bladder stones and more direct access to repair a bladder diverticulum.

For a man with a large prostate, open prostatectomy is a very effective operation. While there is more postoperative pain with this procedure than with a TURP (which causes little if any discomfort), it may be more effective over the long run, as recurrence rates are somewhat lower following open prostatectomy than they are following a TURP. Hospitalization for open prostatectomy lasts about five days.

OTHER PROCEDURES FOR BLOCKAGE:
Transurethral Incision of the Prostate

Transurethral incision of the prostate (TUIP) is an effective endoscopic procedure for relief of *prostatism.* Using either standard high-frequency electrosurgical instruments or *neodinium-YAG* laser, the surgeon creates incisions that open up the bladder neck and prostatic urethra but does not remove tissue from the prostate. Unlike the TURP, TUIP has the advantage of preserving normal outward ejaculation in most patients, and it can be accomplished without overnight hospitalization. Its disadvantages are that it does not remove

FIGURE 7-10
Transurethral Incision of Bladder Neck

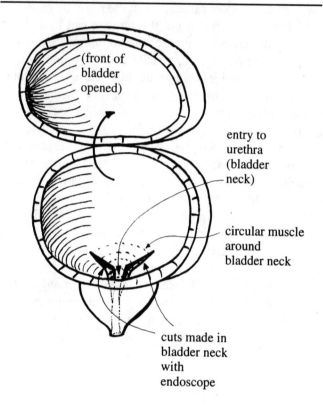

(front of bladder opened)

entry to urethra (bladder neck)

circular muscle around bladder neck

cuts made in bladder neck with endoscope

any tissue that can be examined to check for cancer, and it is slightly less effective in improving urination than TURP. One study showed peak flow rates to average 17.2 milliliters per second after TURP and 12.9 milliliters per second after TUIP. Ninety-eight percent of patients reported overall improvement following TURP, compared with 83 percent following TUIP. For these reasons, the TUIP is a good procedure for younger men with a small but obstructing prostate and not as good when the prostate is larger, median lobe obstruction is present, or cancer is suspected.

A resectoscope is used for this procedure, but the cutting loop is exchanged for a small, wire electrosurgical knife. Electric current allows the knife to cut through the bladder neck and down into the prostatic urethra.

When bleeding vessels have been cauterized and a catheter inserted, the operation is over. The catheter is usually removed the following day.

LASER PROSTATECTOMY

Ever since Luke Skywalker turned on his light saber, popular conception has held that laser energy is the best way to cut. Although this is not the case, laser has its advantages.

Laser light is intensely focused and has unique properties that make it well suited for precise vaporization of tissue. For this reason, medicine has found many uses for lasers, including prostate surgery. Currently two methods are being evaluated for treating prostate blockage with lasers: (1) the transurethral ultrasound-guided laser incision of the prostate (TULIP), and (2) the visually directed laser ablation of the prostate (VLAP). Both procedures require anesthesia.

The TULIP operation uses a laser beam to incise or cut prostate tissue rather than remove it, much like the transurethral incision of the prostate (TUIP). Rather than directing this cutting visually with an endoscope as is done in a TUIP, the TULIP system uses an ultrasound probe placed in the rectum to guide placement of the laser incision. The laser cuts with little or no bleeding, which shortens the associated hospitalization.

The VLAP bears a greater similarity to a TURP. Laser obliteration of the prostate does not cause bleeding and can be done on an outpatient basis. It has fewer risks of immediate surgical complications than a TURP but requires a catheter to be worn for a longer time postoperatively and may be followed by a longer period of irritating symptoms. Furthermore, the recurrence rate for BPH after laser prostatectomy is not known.

For a VLAP, currently the most popular procedure, a standard

FIGURE 7-11
Laser Prostatectomy

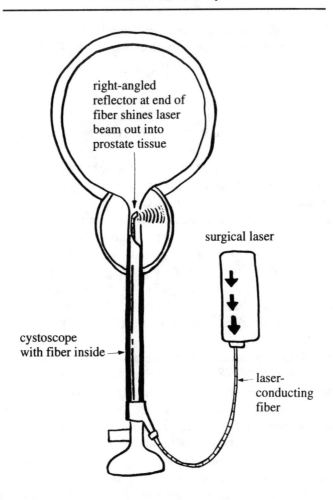

right-angled
reflector at end of
fiber shines laser
beam out into
prostate tissue

surgical laser

cystoscope
with fiber inside →

laser-
conducting
fiber

cystoscope is used. It is equipped with a laser-transmitting fiber, with a reflector at the working end, which deflects the beam out at a right angle from the tip of the scope. With the scope positioned in the prostatic urethra, the right-angle laser beam passes through the urethra and out into the surrounding prostate tissue.

Depending on the type of laser used and the energy delivered, the intense light penetrates into and "cooks" the prostate tissue to a depth of about 1 centimeter, thus *photocoagulating* it. A Foley catheter is then placed, which often must be left in for a week before normal urination resumes. The destroyed tissue is gradually liquified and passed in the urine over the following months. When all photocoagulated tissue has been passed, an open space replaces the former prostatic urethra, much as occurs after a TURP. In a similar fashion to healing after a TURP, a new lining membrane is regenerated to pave the path from the bladder to the urethra.

Neither laser procedure removes tissue for pathologic examination, which would allow a pathologist to check for cancer. Although the preliminary results are exciting, we do not have the number of cases or long-term follow-up necessary to confirm the relationship laser surgery will have to conventional surgery. We do not know the recurrence rate for BPH after laser prostatectomy. Until these data are available, we should view laser prostatectomy as a promising technique in the early stage of development.

BALLOON DILATION

In this procedure, a specially designed catheter with a strong balloon at the end is positioned in the prostatic urethra either by X-ray or by direct vision through a scope. Pressurized inflation of the balloon stretches the urethra within the prostate from its normal diameter (close to that of a pencil) to that of the thumb.

Although balloon dilation is a minimally invasive technique with little blood loss, its long-term effect is questionable. Although several studies have shown symptomatic improvement in the months following balloon dilation, it appears that the improvement doesn't last long. One study found the long-term outcome in patients undergoing balloon dilation to be the same as in patients who had undergone cystoscopy alone, without balloon dilation. The consensus is that this procedure represents a delaying tactic for one too ill to have surgery, rather than a definitive treatment for BPH.

INTRAURETHRAL STENTS

This experimental method is based on placing a small self-retaining tube within the compressed prostatic urethra. The tube, or stent, holds the urethra open and allows urine to pass through more freely. These tubes are made of wire coils or mesh, which permits them to become embedded or incorporated into the prostatic urethra and covered with the usual urethral lining. Insertion is a short procedure and in many cases relieves urinary retention; however, its drawbacks include infection, movement of the stent, discomfort, and difficulty catheterizing the patient. At present, there has been insufficient clinical study of this method to indicate its value and long-term risks.

HEATING THE PROSTATE

Doctors have long recommended hot baths for prostate inflammation, recognizing that application of heat can reduce some symptoms. Cancer research has also found a beneficial effect of heat on tumor reduction, and because of this, microwave techniques were developed to heat tumors locally. This technology has been extended to the patient with BPH.

Systems providing *microwave heating* through either a probe placed in the rectum, or a catheter placed in the urethra, have been used. The transurethral approach appears to be most effective in heating the prostate. Temperatures 20 to 40 percent above normal body temperature can be safely produced in the prostate by a microwave antenna in a special catheter. Water cooling through the catheter protects the urethra, and a rectal temperature probe monitors the dispersed heat to ensure safety. Pilot studies have shown improvement of 50 to 80 percent in symptoms. One study showed that 40 percent of a group of patients using catheters for retention were able to resume urination after microwave hyperthemia therapy. This approach is appealing, as it is a nonsurgical forty-five-minute outpatient procedure that does not require anesthesia. As is the case with most other new emerging treatments, however, we do not have a long track record to study. Until sufficient data are available, the role of hyperthermia in treating BPH will be uncertain.

CANCER SURGERY

Operations done on patients with prostate cancer are intended to either be *curative* (eliminate the cancer) or *palliative* (improve the patient's condition but not cure the cancer). For example, a patient with a very large prostate tumor may suffer from symptoms of blockage. If because of his age or advanced tumor stage he is not a candidate for curative removal of the prostate, he may benefit from a TURP. This endoscopic procedure will not cure the cancer, but it will make urination much easier. Similarly, a bilateral orchiectomy does not cure prostate cancer in a man with metastatic disease, but it usually improves his condition dramatically.

Surgery for the Cure of Prostate Cancer

In chapter 6 we discussed how surgical removal of the cancerous prostate can produce prolonged disease-free survival in men with cancer confined to the prostate. Since their disease-free survival following surgery is equivalent to the survival that men of similar age would experience if they didn't have prostate cancer, it is appropriate to say that for men in this most favorable group, surgery can cure cancer.

Surgical Staging: A Prerequisite to Curative Cancer Surgery

Since the earliest spread from prostate cancer is to the surrounding lymph nodes, showing that the lymph nodes are free from the disease is considered sufficient proof that the cancer has not spread. As reviewed in chapter 6, nonsurgical imaging tests are not reliable enough to make this determination. Since surgical removal of the prostate for cure succeeds only when the cancer is localized to the prostate, surgical determination of lymph node status is required first.

The majority of surgeons perform a *lymphadenectomy* (removal of the lymph nodes) through a six-inch vertical lower abdominal incision. After a pathologist has examined the nodes using a *frozen section technique* (microscopic slices of the nodes are reviewed while the patient is still on the operating table, which takes five to ten minutes) and found no evidence of cancer, the surgeon can perform a *radical retropubic prostatectomy* through the same incision. This type of lymphadenectomy takes about thirty minutes and involves removing the lymph nodes from around the major vessels and nerves adjacent to the prostate (see figure 6–4). Less commonly, endoscopic instruments are used to puncture the peritoneal (abdominal) cavity and perform lymphadenectomy. This technique of *laparoscopic lymphadenectomy* uses four puncture wounds of about one-half inch each, rather than a single vertical incision. If examination of the lymph nodes shows no cancer, the patient is scheduled for surgery (through a standard incision) at a later date.

Although laparoscopic lymphadenectomy involves a smaller incision, the procedure is performed within the intestinal or abdominal cavity, in contrast to standard lymphadenectomy, which is *extraperitoneal* (performed outside the abdominal cavity). Operating within the abdominal cavity increases the risk of bowel obstruction or injury, which is quite low with the standard extraperitoneal approach. The laparoscopic procedure takes two to three hours. For these reasons, it may be the best choice for that small group of patients who have elected radiation therapy for cure but who have a significant chance of positive lymph nodes. Patients with a PSA greater than 20, or high-grade cancer (Gleason 8 or higher), have a greater chance of lymph node involvement and benefit from accurate surgical staging. Radiation therapy is ineffective if the nodes are positive.

Prostate Removal for Cancer

Radical prostatectomy refers to the removal of the entire prostate, including the seminal vesicles and a small cuff of attached bladder neck. This is distinct from simple prostatectomy, wherein the obstructing inner part of the prostate is shelled out, leaving the remainder of the prostate intact. Simple prostatectomy is an operation for BPH, not cancer.

Radical prostatectomy can be performed in two ways: radical *retropubic* prostatectomy, through a six-inch vertical incision between the umbilicus and pubic bone, and radical *perineal* prostatectomy, done through an incision in the perineum, between the anus and the scrotum. Because it allows concomitant staging and lymph node dissection, the retropubic approach is more common. Depending on the size of the tumor, it is often possible to preserve the nerves that produce erection, allowing the majority of sexually active men with a small prostate tumor to remain so after surgery. Temporary urinary incontinence is common after radical prostatectomy, although fewer than 5 percent of patients suffer permanently. Most surgical patients will require transfusion. If the patient's own blood is banked during the weeks before surgery, the use of blood from anonymous donors is reduced. Hospitalization generally lasts for five to seven days.

After the major pelvic vessels have been exposed and the lymphadenectomy completed, the front of the prostate comes into view, between the floor of the pelvis and the bladder. The first step in a radical retropubic prostatectomy is to remove the lower end, or *apex,* of the prostate from its attachment to the urethra as it exits through the muscle floor of the pelvis and runs down into the penis. This requires detaching a large collection of veins that enter the top of the prostate from the penis, cutting the urethra as it leaves the lower part of the prostate, and dividing a thin muscle between the urethra and the rectum.

At this point, the paired nerves that run next to the prostate as they travel down to the erection mechanism in the penis can be seen. When tumor size permits, one or both sides can be saved as the prostate is lifted upward, which can preserve the ability for erection in many patients (see also chapter 8). The prostate (with seminal vesicles) is then detached from the bladder and removed.

After the prostate has been removed, it is necessary to narrow the bladder neck so it fits the cut end of the urethra. The two structures are then sewn together over a catheter.

TABLE 7-1
Prostate Operations

Operation	Indications	Risks and complications	Results	Advantages/ disadvantages	Recovery time	Total cost
Transurethral incision of prostate (TUIP)	Bladder blockage, smaller prostate, younger men	Bleeding, stricture, may cause retrograde ejaculation	Good improvement in flow rates	Short hospitalization, less chance of retrograde ejaculation/Blockage may recur in time, no tissue removed for biopsy	1 week	$3,000
Transurethral resection of prostate (TURP)	Bladder blockage, retention	Bleeding, stricture, impotence	Excellent improvement in flow rates	No incision, most reliable operation for blockage/Retrograde ejaculation, hospitalization required	2 weeks	$4,000
Laser ablation	Same as TURP	Stricture, impotence, prolonged catheter use, failure to relieve blockage	Good—Fair (short-term), long-term unknown	No hospitalization/No tissue removed for biopsy	1–4 weeks	$3,000

Balloon dilation	Bladder blockage	Bleeding, failure	Fair: short-term, Poor: long-term	No hospitalization/No tissue removed, effect doesn't last long	1 week	$2,000
Suprapubic prostatectomy	Bladder blockage, bladder stones or diverticulum, large prostate	Bleeding, stricture, impotence	Excellent improvement in flow rates	Good when large stones or diverticulum present/Longer hospitalization, more pain	3–4 weeks	$7,000
Retropubic prostatectomy	Bladder blockage, large prostate	Bleeding, stricture, impotence	Excellent improvement in flow rates	Best method for large prostates/Longer hospitalization	3–4 weeks	$7,000
Radical prostatectomy	Localized prostate cancer	Bleeding, stricture, impotence, incontinence	High chance for cure with early cancer	Best 15-year survival figures for localized cancer/Potential effect on erections, slight chance of incontinence	6 weeks	$15,000

Before the incision is closed, a drain is inserted. This is a soft rubber tube that sits outside the bladder and urethra in the pelvis, allowing the urinary leakage or ooze of blood that occurs in the first day or two to exit rather than build up inside.

Hospitalization for this procedure usually lasts five to seven days. At the time of discharge, the patient is sent home with a catheter still in, connected to a leg bag. This allows the patient to walk and undertake other activities in normal clothing, which is encouraged postoperatively. The catheter is removed three weeks after surgery in the doctor's office; the procedure is not painful. Most patients experience some urinary leakage requiring the use of pads for the first week or two after the catheter comes out. Regaining urinary control can often take a month or two. When a nerve-sparing operation is done, return of erections can take up to one year.

FIGURE 7-12
Radical Retropubic Prostatectomy

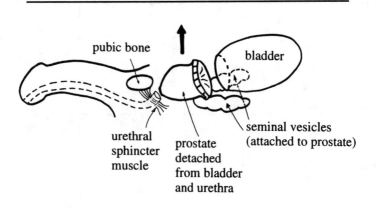

FIGURE 7-13
Radical Retropubic Prostatectomy—Closing

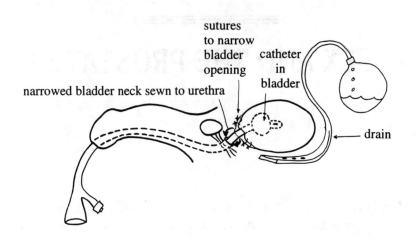

sutures
to narrow
bladder
opening

catheter
in
bladder

narrowed bladder neck sewn to urethra

drain

Chapter 8

═══════════════════

SEX AND THE PROSTATE

I didn't know Russell well, so I might have thought he talked a bigger game than he played. I would have been wrong. He was well into his seventies, but he looked younger and had twinkling eyes that seemed to follow the nurses. He also had a catheter because his bladder was blocked up with BPH.

His daughter told me he feared prostate surgery would "ruin his manhood." He had been avoiding it until his Central American housekeeper ran off. The daughter related how difficult it had been to retain a housekeeper for her father—he chased them all. He ended up having a TURP, which didn't change anything except to rid him of the catheter. I didn't get a chance to talk to his daughter after surgery, as his new housekeeper brought him in for the postoperative visit. From what I could tell, they had already become quite friendly.

The prostate gland belongs to one of the complex systems that contribute to a man's sexuality. Disorders of this organ and their treatment may affect sexual activity, although the body's ability to recover is remarkable in men unwilling to relinquish the fundamental roots of intimacy.

Sexual interest is constant to the point of distraction in young men: sex becomes a preoccupation, and performance is unwavering even in the most adverse circumstances. By the time the forties hit, men may note that interest—and, to a lesser extent, capacity—vary from day to day and week to week. Even though the pleasure of sex remains unchanged, desire is more affected by various physical and mental rhythms, and the business of daily life more frequently intrudes into primary biologic functions.

Awareness of the ebb and flow of bodily rhythms is beneficial, and men should tolerate some amount of variation in sexual capacity. Of course, lessened desire and borderline performance should not be sought after, but some appreciation of the natural variability of personal response should be cultivated. However, if sexual capacity falls far enough below expectation to produce frustration, or disharmony in a relationship, something is wrong. If this condition persists, medical assistance should be sought.

Impotence means the inability to obtain and/or keep an erection hard enough for adequate sexual activity. Currently, the term *erectile dysfunction* is preferred, as it is more descriptive and less demeaning. Although erectile dysfunction is only one facet of male sexual malfunction, it is the most disturbing symptom and the one most commonly responsible for clinic visits. Surveys have shown that erectile problems are the most common complaints of men attending sexual dysfunction clinics, and are some of the biggest fears of men with prostate problems.

WHAT IS SEX?

Dumb question! If you have to ask, you will never understand the answer. Actually, we are looking beyond its biological role as a preferred method of reproduction and beyond its power as a profound influence on our relationships with others. Relationships reflect back an interpreted version of ourselves, crucial to the formation of a self-image. When anything goes wrong with sex, it shakes the established image a man has about himself. When women have trouble sexually, they often wonder about the relationship; when men have trouble, they wonder about themselves.

Most major causes of erectile dysfunction have a physical basis or contributing physical factors. Identifying them helps, as you can worry about something specific and correctable and not concentrate on your "failure" as a person. Of course, solving sexual problems does mean having to take a look at our ideas about ourselves, but that's about enough psychology for now.

WHERE TO START

Perhaps we should start in seventh grade, before the days of baggy pants, when unstoppable erections first began to be a source of embarrassment. Or maybe with the first date, the first hug or close encounter with someone who had a powerful effect on you.

Narrowing the view to erection, ejaculation, and the biology responsible for these processes will provide an easier way to connect sexual success and failure with the prostate and its associated plumbing. It may make sex appear well defined—a mechanical and predictable activity, which it isn't. Nonetheless, there is an underlying order to the way it all works, and the temporary reduction of a complex process to an oversimplified mechanism increases understanding.

HOW ERECTIONS WORK

Men equate sex with getting a hard erection, having intercourse, and ejaculating. Women certainly take the above into account, but their picture is bigger, involving other factors. Despite the differences in perspective, normal erectile function is central to most varieties of sexual expression in men.

There are two chambers, called the *corpora cavernosa,* that inflate with blood, become firm, and cause the penis to get hard.

These paired cigar-shaped cylinders are the "erection mechanism," and most of our ideas about the mechanics of erection can be traced to their function. The outer wall of the corpora cavernosa is a thick sheet of connective tissue called the *tunica albuginea.* This material forms the wall of what acts like a balloon but shows differences in behavior when compared with a thin sheet of rubber. It extends, or stretches with little resistance or effort, until its maximal

FIGURE 8-1
Erection Chambers

corpora cavernosa

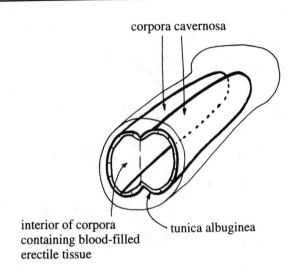

interior of corpora
containing blood-filled
erectile tissue

tunica albuginea

dimensions are reached, then pulls tight and will expand no further. This size limitation that is built into the "balloon wall" is what produces hardness with inflation—if it simply continued to stretch like rubber, the penis would get bigger and bigger as blood filled it but would not become hard.

Enclosed within the tunica albuginea is a specialized spongy tissue that can fill with blood during erection, expand, and stretch the tunica to the point of hardness. This internal erectile tissue is made of little blood spaces, called *sinusoids,* that are fed by arteries and emptied by veins.

The walls of the sinusoids contain muscle, similar to the coating of an artery. Appropriate nerve stimulation causes relaxation of this muscle, which causes the arteries to open and the walls of the sinusoids to become more lax. Increasing blood flow through the dilated arteries fills and expands the relaxed sinusoids. Enlargement of the sinusoids as they fill is the first step in inflation of the penis

FIGURE 8-2
Erectile Tissue—Sinusoids

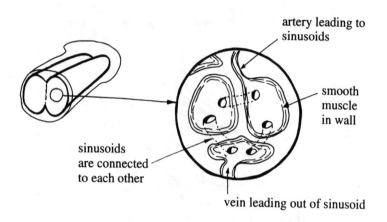

artery leading to
sinusoids

smooth
muscle
in wall

sinusoids
are connected
to each other

vein leading out of sinusoid

to cause an erection, but it is not sufficient to complete or maintain the process. For full erection to be reached, the sinusoid walls must relax enough to allow the entire mass of sinusoidal tissue to expand and press on the surrounding tunica albuginea, which when stretched to its inherent size is quite unyielding. The veins that drain blood out of the sinusoids run under the tunica and are squashed shut as dilated erectile tissue expands against the unyielding tunica.

If open, these veins would act like holes in a balloon, which would defeat efforts to blow it up. Closure of these veins by the mechanism just described permits complete and sustained inflation of the corpora, stretching the tunica to its size limit, where it becomes firm.

Erection takes place when signals traveling into the corpora cavernosa through the *cavernous nerves* cause release of special chemicals, or *neurotransmitters,* that relax the muscles of the sinusoid and artery wall. Research suggests the chemical released in this process may be *nitric oxide.* There are drugs that mimic the muscle-relaxing effects of naturally occurring neurotransmitters, and they can be used in the treatment of erectile problems.

Figure 8-3
Blood Trapping Mechanism in Erectile Chambers

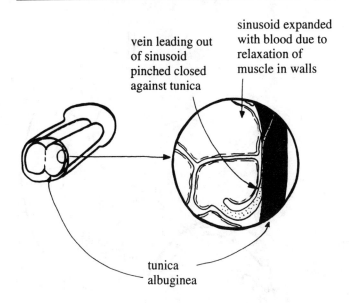

vein leading out
of sinusoid
pinched closed
against tunica

sinusoid expanded
with blood due to
relaxation of
muscle in walls

tunica
albuginea

The cavernous nerves enter the corpora cavernosa just below the prostate gland. These nerves run from the lower spinal cord down into the penis and right next to the prostate. They come particularly close together near its apex, or lower end. The cavernous nerves are paired, running on the right and left sides of the pelvis. When both nerves are damaged, erection will not occur. Injury to these nerves from surgery or radiation therapy can cause impotence. Experience has shown that if only one side is injured, functional erections may continue. For this reason, and to avoid cutting too close to a cancerous prostate, surgeons may be able to save only the right or the left cavernous nerve during radical prostatectomy, in some cases. Although this often results in salvage of a patient's erections, the best results occur when both nerves can be saved.

There are several ways signals can be sent down the cavernous nerves to turn on an erection. Physical sensations from sensory

FIGURE 8-4
Cavernous Nerves

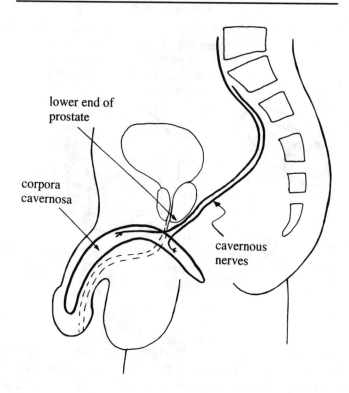

lower end of
prostate

corpora
cavernosa

cavernous
nerves

nerves in the genital area can connect with and activate the cavernous nerves in the lower spinal cord without passing through the
brain. Of course, erotic sights and thoughts must send signals from
the brain down the spinal cord to affect cavernous nerve activity and
cause erections. This means that an intact spinal cord is required to
"think up" an erection, but also that genital touch alone can cause
a reflex, or automatic, erection in someone with a spinal cord injury
above the level where the genital sensory nerves and cavernous
nerves connect.

EJACULATION

Continued genital stimulation culminates in the forceful expulsion of semen. *Ejaculation* involves a different set of nerves than erection, so that erection may occur without ejaculation and vice versa. When erection is present, ejaculation triggers a neurochemical change that ends the relaxation of the artery and sinusoidal muscle, causing the erection to go down. The effects of this reaction takes some time to wear off. During this time, or *refractory period,* the sinusoidal smooth muscle cannot be made to relax, so the erection

FIGURE 8-5
Ejaculation

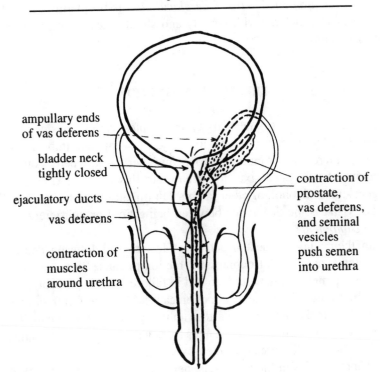

ampullary ends
of vas deferens

bladder neck
tightly closed

ejaculatory ducts

vas deferens

contraction of
muscles
around urethra

contraction of
prostate,
vas deferens,
and seminal
vesicles
push semen
into urethra

cannot be reestablished. This period may extend for minutes, in a young man, to a day or more in an older man.

Ejaculation occurs when sufficient nerve stimulation causes the seminal vesicles and ampullary ends of the vas deferens to contract, expelling semen through the ejaculatory ducts into the prostatic urethra. This is accompanied by contractions of muscle within the prostate gland and bladder neck.

With the upper urethra full of semen (the usual amount is about one tablespoon), and the ring-like bladder neck tightly contracted and closed, semen has nowhere to go but down the urethra and out of the penis.

As the seminal discharge follows this route, it is forcibly propelled by rhythmic contractions of the muscles around the urethra at the base of the penis. If the bladder neck is unable to close because of surgical changes or drug effects, ejaculation back into the bladder may occur. So-called *retrograde ejaculation* is not harmful, but it can present problems with fertility and slightly alters the sensation of ejaculation.

ERECTILE DYSFUNCTION

The frequency of sexual activity in couples varies considerably. More than 70 percent of men between ages twenty and thirty report having intercourse from two to four times per week, whereas only 6 percent of men aged sixty to seventy are this active. Extreme fatigue, stress, alcohol, or other factors can impair erections in normal men. What is the difference between being tired or indifferent and being *impotent?*

In their study of sexual activity, Masters and Johnson defined impotence as enough trouble with erection to cause 25 percent of a man's attempts at intercourse to end in failure. This is probably a bit too simplified. If erectile dysfunction causes a man to fail frequently enough to make him or his partner unhappy, he has a problem. The prevalence of such difficulty ranges from less than 7 percent in men under forty to 30 percent in men over sixty.

Abnormalities in blood vessels, nerves, or hormones can prevent a man from getting a functional, rigid erection or can make erection impossible to sustain. Erection requires an increase in blood flow to the penis, so any disorder that affects the arteries may impair erection. Smoking, as well as atherosclerosis—the same hardening of the arteries that can cause heart disease and poor circulation—can do this. In addition to increased blood inflow, getting an erection requires the veins that let blood out of the corpora cavernosa to close down and reduce blood outflow. If the veins "leak" and let blood out, keeping a hard erection can be difficult. Loss of elasticity in the connective tissue supporting the veins or within the erectile tissue itself, due to diabetes or other disorders, can inhibit the way veins close during erection.

Damage to the nerves that carry sensation from the penis or to those automatic nerves that regulate blood flow changes within the penis can cause erectile failure. Diabetes, spinal cord disease, or trauma can have this effect. Very specific nerve pathways must be altered; common back strains or injuries, even those involving a "bad disc," usually do not affect erection. Injury to the cavernous nerves adjacent to the prostate, occurring with radiation or surgery for prostate cancer, can be responsible for erectile dysfunction.

Testosterone plays an important role in regulating sexual desire and affects erection as well. Decreased testosterone levels from a variety of causes can produce sexual apathy or erectile dysfunction. Not all men who undergo orchiectomy or other equivalent hormone deprivation therapy for metastatic prostate cancer become impotent, but this change has a profound effect on the quality of erection and sexual desire.

Genital discomfort can inhibit erection. When bacterial prostatitis produces perineal or penile pain, or makes ejaculation painful, reduction in desire and erection may be the body's temporary adjustment. Chronic disorders may introduce unpredictability to erectile responses, but they often involve psychologic factors as well.

Major relationship problems, anxiety, or depression can have a negative impact on sexual function. While the cause of erectile dysfunction in this setting has usually been termed "psychologic," the subtle changes in body chemistry that occur with severe anxiety, for example, may retard erection by interfering with the physical changes required to relax arterial and sinusoidal smooth muscle. Erectile dysfunction has traditionally been divided into *organic*, which has physical causes, and *psychogenic*, which has mental causes. In the past, most cases of erectile dysfunction were thought to be psychogenic. Current research has shown that the opposite is true—most patients with erectile dysfunction have a contributing physical cause as well. Because of the seamless interaction of physical and psychological factors in sexual response, malfunction usually involves several different factors.

Prescription drugs can interfere with erection and produce impotence. In one study, drugs were responsible for 25 percent of impotence cases seen in a sexual dysfunction clinic. With the central role played by blood vessel changes in erection, it is not surprising that high blood pressure medications, which target blood vessel behavior, commonly produce problems with erection. A great variety of high blood pressure medications are available. Drugs that directly affect arterial muscle, blood-converting enzymes, calcium channels, or increased fluid and salt output (diuretics) are least likely to cause impotence. Drugs known as beta blockers, and drugs acting on the autonomic nervous system's control of blood vessel dilation, are more likely to produce problems. Patients with established high blood pressure may have damage to small vessels, which are less able to transmit the high flow required for erections when their blood pressure has been reduced by medication. Tranquilizers and antidepressants can cause erectile dysfunction, either by reduction in libido or by direct interference with critical nerve function.

Recreational drugs are also capable of impairing erection. In the Masters and Johnson study, alcohol use was one of the top causes of erectile dysfunction. Marijuana may depress testosterone levels and have a negative effect on erection when used for a long time. Cocaine can impair erection by causing *vasoconstriction* (narrowing of blood vessels) or reduced libido.

THE PROSTATE AND SEXUAL FUNCTION

Most forms of sexual impairment have been attributed at one time or another to abnormalities of the prostate gland, perhaps because of its central role in a man's sexual physiology. The effects of sexual excess or deprivation were popular themes with authors of a previous era, who described how men could "strain" the gland by having too much sex or too little. Before reviewing some of the sexual effects the prostate can cause, these should be put into perspective. Data from clinics treating men for sexual dysfunction show that prostate abnormalities are a minor contributor to serious sexual impairment such as impotence. Except for aggressive curative therapy for early prostate cancer, most disorders of this gland and their treatments will not substantially impair a man's ability to have intercourse.

Sexual activity may decrease somewhat with aging, during the time when many men become aware of urinary symptoms due to prostate enlargement. The two processes may take place in parallel, but this does not imply that one causes the other. There is some reassurance in seeing the processes of sexual and urinary slowdown as minor adjustments, not unstoppable progressive trends. Men do not become impotent just by getting older, and most men's urinary symptoms due to prostate enlargement will not progress to the point of needing surgery.

Pain with Ejaculation

Pain with ejaculation is usually caused by inflammation within the prostate. This is a chemical and cellular response that may be caused by infection or by other less easily identified factors. Minor discomfort may be noted with ejaculation if it follows a long period of sexual abstinence, and this has no consequence. More significant pain with ejaculation usually responds to treatment of prostate inflammation or infection. This condition can cause temporary avoidance or reduction in desire, which gradually clears up with resolution of the underlying cause.

Premature Ejaculation

Premature ejaculation, or the inability to delay climax until the appropriate time, can also be caused by prostate inflammation. The nerve stimulation caused by inflammation can add to the sexual stimulation usually responsible for ejaculation and cause climax to occur with less sexual stimulation. This will resolve with treatment of prostatitis when that is the contributing cause. Some men suffer from a more serious problem, which may begin with the onset of sexual activity and persist through adult life. Long-standing and persistent premature ejaculation is probably not caused by prostate disease. It can be treated by sexual therapists, who may instruct the patient to withdraw when climax nears, and compress the junction of the shaft and head of the penis with the thumb and forefinger for a few moments until the feeling passes. Drug therapy with terazosin or metoclopramide has also been used successfully in men with persistent premature ejaculation.

Bloody Ejaculation

Bloody ejaculation, or *hematospermia,* is alarming to see, although it rarely implies serious problems. When inflammation of the prostate ducts or the lining of the seminal vesicles produces blood vessel changes that permit bleeding into the channels of the semen delivery mechanism, ejaculation can be pink, bright red, or rust-colored. Blood in the urine increases the likelihood that this problem has a serious cause, and prostate cancer must be considered. If urinalysis shows the urine to be clear of blood cells, the rectal exam result is normal, and the PSA level is normal, bloody ejaculation can be safely ignored until it goes away on its own. On those rare occasions when it persists for months, short therapy with an estrogen-like hormone will usually stop it.

Retrograde Ejaculation

Retrograde ejaculation is passage of the semen back into the bladder rather than out the end of the penis. It occurs with the sensation of climax, which may be altered slightly, but there is lack of any visible discharge. The semen mixes with urine in the bladder and is discharged the next time urination occurs. As has been discussed previously, alteration of the bladder neck by surgery or drugs is the usual cause.

FIGURE 8-6
Retrograde Ejaculation

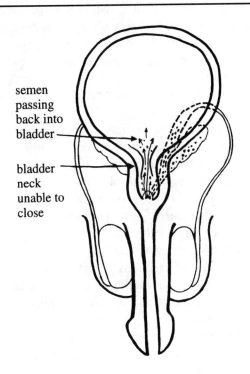

semen
passing
back into
bladder —

bladder —
neck
unable to
close

Sexual Overindulgence

Multiple ejaculations occurring over a period of hours may cause a lingering discomfort at the base of the penis or in the perineum. This discomfort, probably due to repeatedly forceful muscular contractions in and around the prostate, is self-limited and will disappear in a short time.

Sexual Abstinence

Long periods without ejaculation can cause symptoms within the prostate similar to those seen in nonbacterial prostatitis. These symptoms may be more pronounced in men who experience frequent sexual stimulation but not the culmination and release of climax and ejaculation. Such "congestion" within the prostate was once thought to be the source of a variety of sexual problems. There is no current evidence that unfulfilled desire or its physiologic consequences lead to BPH, prostate cancer, or other problems.

Impotence

Temporary loss of erections, or inability to maintain enough hardness for intercourse, can occur with infection or inflammation of the prostate. Prolonged soaks in a hot tub, an often-recommended treatment for prostatic inflammation, also has an inhibiting effect on erection. These factors will not produce chronic, persistent, or long-lasting alteration of erection, however.

Radiation therapy for prostate cancer affects the cavernous nerves, but only 40 percent of patients who have been sexually active prior to therapy report loss of erections with treatment. Although there may be some alteration in the quality of erections following therapy, at least half of these patients will be able to continue sexual activity without undue interference.

Radical prostatectomy for cancer can be done using a technique that avoids nerve damage in patients with small tumors. The results with so-called "nerve-sparing prostatectomy" are related to the patient's age and preoperative sexual activity. In young, sexually active patients with very small tumors, the outcome clearly surpasses that obtained with radiation therapy. Among all men undergoing the operation, the results are more similar: slightly more than half of the patients undergoing nerve-sparing radical prostatectomy will obtain usable, reliable erections postoperatively. The recovery period for erections is quite prolonged—up to one year.

In general, prostate disorders do not make their appearance in the form of impotence. Erectile failure can be the first indication of other serious disorders, however. For this reason, men with new or persistent erectile difficulties should be evaluated medically. A history and physical examination is a mandatory first step.

Following this, a few tests are routinely recommended. Measurement of serum testosterone levels can identify hormonal causes of sexual dysfunction, which are often present in a man with low desire. Injection of a medication that relaxes the muscle of the sinusoids and blood vessels within the penis is helpful in testing the vascular system. When this injection produces an erection that is close to normal, serious arterial disease is quite unlikely. This test is often supplemented by a measurement of the blood pressure in the penis after injection, using a small blood pressure cuff and a sensitive, electronically amplified stethoscope. The blood pressure thus measured in the penis should be at least 80 percent of the routine blood pressure taken at the arm. This percentage, known as the *penile-brachial index,* is helpful in identifying underlying blood vessel disease. When it is well below 80 percent, other blood vessel studies are indicated to evaluate flow and function in major arteries. When appropriate, a blood glucose test is useful to check for diabetes, since this fairly common condition is an important contributing cause of erectile dysfunction.

In the past, the importance of distinguishing psychogenic erectile dysfunction from organic erectile dysfunction was emphasized. While these are clearly meaningful categories, they were most important when the only treatment option available was major surgery. As there are now treatment options that may be appropriate for either group, this difference may not be so critical. Moreover, it is now recognized that serious erectile dysfunction frequently involves both psychological and physical malfunction.

Evaluation of impotence should be considered as *goal directed* by the patient: the testing that is done should be determined by the length the patient wants to go to solve his problem. If he is content with nonsurgical therapy, the testosterone and glucose measurements, followed by the injection test, are probably sufficient evaluation. If he wishes to proceed with surgery, and the evidence suggests that psychological factors are stronger than physical disorders, monitoring of erections during sleep may be helpful. This test, *nocturnal tumescence monitoring,* is a way of measuring whether any erectile activity occurs during sleep. Normal men— even normal men with psychologically impaired erectile function— experience nighttime erections. In men with nerve injury, blood

FIGURE 8-7
Testing Blood Flow into Penis

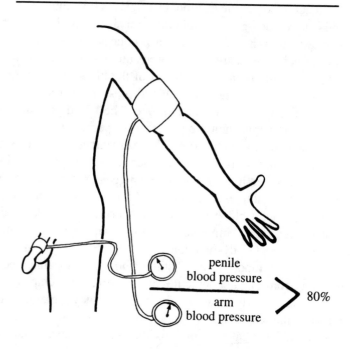

vessel disease, or other physical impediment, nocturnal erections are reduced.

Detailed testing of corpora cavernosa function by monitoring pressures during controlled fluid infusion is a research-oriented approach that is not necessary in the majority of men with impotence. This type of study, and perhaps *angiography,* or X-rays of penile blood vessels, may be necessary in a highly select group of men with impotence following blood vessel injury.

TREATMENT OF ERECTILE DYSFUNCTION

Evaluation of the impotent man may reveal specific medical or psychological abnormalities. Unfortunately, treatment directed at these specific abnormalities will restore erections in relatively few situations. Impotence associated with abnormally low serum testosterone levels will usually respond to hormone replacement. Diabetes is a far more common hormone problem producing impotence, but its control with medications or hormone replacement (insulin) may not restore erections. Injury to specific penile arteries (by pelvic fracture, for example) may produce impotence that can be corrected by a meticulous bypass procedure. Impotence due to hardening or obliteration of major abdominal or pelvic arteries will not usually be corrected by surgical bypass. Psychotherapy has been reported to be helpful in psychologically impaired men with normal bodily function, but there are no good numerical data on the outcomes or successes of this approach.

More men with impotence have physical causes than primary psychological causes. Unfortunately, the complexity of these causes, and the subtlety of their effects on the penis, frustrate efforts to fine-tune the body and fix the penis as a consequence. For this reason, advances in treatment for erectile dysfunction have been directed primarily at the erectile mechanism within the penis itself.

Returning for a moment to the basics, erection can be produced by causing the corpora cavernosa to expand until its outer shell, the tunica albuginea, is pulled taut. This can be accomplished medically by inducing the corpora to fill with blood, or surgically by filling the corpora with implanted cylinders that stretch the tunica.

Drugs

Some drugs start out as folk or tribal medicine, graduating to prescription status when scientific investigation confirms their worth. One example is *yohimbine,* an alkaloid substance extracted from the bark of an African tree, *Corynanthe johimbi.* Teas or other preparations of the bark were said to have aphrodisiac properties. Laboratory studies identified the active principle as the yohimbine alkaloid, which works by stopping certain nerves from causing blood vessels to constrict or close down. The result is dilation or opening of blood vessels, with increased blood flow in the genital region. Clinical studies have shown more than a placebo effect, with about 60 percent of men reporting improved erections.

TABLE 8–1
Impotence Treatment

Rx	Indications	Risks, Side Effects	Results	Advantages/ Disadvantages	Cost
Yohimbine	Partial erections, difficulty sustaining	Nervousness, flushing	About 60% of men improve	Inexpensive, easy to take/Ineffective	$25/mo
Injection therapy	Absent or inadequate erections, difficulty sustaining	Priapism (prolonged erection), scarring of erectile bodies	Good results in about 85%	Usually very effective for severe erectile dysfunction/Requires injection, may cause priapism	$35/mo
Vacuum erection device	Absent or inadequate erections, difficulty sustaining	Bruising of penis	Good results in 80–90%	No medication required, no danger of priapism/Cumbersome setup, can't use for more than 20-30 minutes	$350

Implant surgery	Absent or inadequate erections	Requires anesthesia, mechanical malfunction, infection or erosion (wearing through tissue), pain	Patient and partner satisfied about 90% of the time	Very effective—near normal erection/ Expensive; possibility of medical complications	$6,500
Counseling	Quality of erection dependent on partner	Preoccupation with problem	Fair improvement in men with primary psychological problems	Often increases communication with partner/May not work	$250/mo
Hormone treatment	Hormone deficiency	Too much testosterone could activate an occult prostate cancer	Good results if hormone deficiency present	Treatment of choice for low-hormone state/ Usually applicable— hormone deficiency is rare cause of impotence	$125/mo
Penile vascular surgery	Specific arterial injury, usually due to trauma (not hardening of arteries)	Requires anesthesia, failure	Fair results in very specific situations	May restore erections after pelvic injury/ Only applicable in rare cases—not suited for most cases	$8,000

As a prescription medication it is known as *yohimbine hydrochloride* and is given as a 5-milligram pill three times a day. Its potential side effects include flushing of the skin and nervousness. Yohimbine hydrochloride is present in varying amounts in *Yohimbe,* a bark extract that can be purchased at health food stores. These preparations vary in makeup, with different batches of the same product or different pills from the same bottle showing considerable variation in strength. A recent study found that treatment with the prescription variety was slightly lower in cost than the natural bark extract.

The same drugs that were used to test erection by relaxing the muscle of the penile sinusoids and arteries can be effective as treatment for impotence. Papaverine, Regitine, prostaglandin E_1, or a combination of these agents have powerful muscle-relaxing effects within the penis. By loosening the muscles that keep the sinusoids contracted down, and dilating arteries with resulting increasing blood flow into the penis, they mimic the initiation of erection by cavernous nerve signals. Since the injections cause the same effect as normal nerve input and are powerful enough to open even diseased arteries, they can successfully restore erections to men with neurologic or vascular abnormalities.

Although injections can produce erection by bypassing a number of abnormalities, they must be given every time an erection is desired. A spot on the side of the penis is selected and is poked with a very fine (30 gauge) needle. This sounds intolerable but in fact is not painful. Within ten to twenty minutes of injection, erection ensues and usually lasts about one hour. In some cases, use of injections over many months may produce improvement in a man's natural or spontaneous erection. The disadvantages of this method are its lack of spontaneity, the supplies required, and the possible adverse effects upon the penis. These can include scarring due to repeat injection that can produce irreversible deformity of the penis, or prolonged erections that require medical attention. *Priapism,* or erection that persists in the absence of desire, can damage the erectile mechanism if allowed to persist for more than five or six hours. Fortunately, this condition rarely follows injection therapy, occurring in about one out of two hundred patients. When treated promptly with the proper medications, it is easily reversible. Some evidence of scarring within the penis is seen in 10 to 20 percent of men on long-term injection therapy, but it usually does not produce significant deformity.

Pressure Effects

A reasonable semblance of an erection can be brought on without drugs or surgery by increasing the pressure within the corpora cavernosum relative to the outside. This is accomplished not by pumping up the pressure inside but by reducing the pressure outside the penis. *Vacuum erection devices* cause the corpora to fill with enough blood to stretch the tunica albuginea and simulate an erection by creating a vacuum outside the penis. A small chamber similar to a jelly jar is placed over the penis and pressed into the skin around its base to create an effective pressure seal. Pumping the air out of the jar with a small attached vacuum pump pulls blood into the interior of the penis.

FIGURE 8-8
Vacuum Erection Device

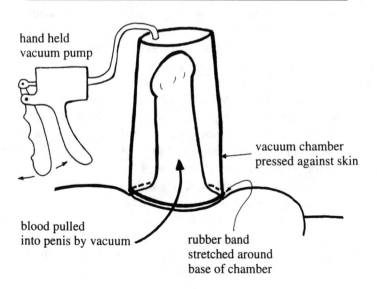

hand held
vacuum pump

vacuum chamber
pressed against skin

blood pulled
into penis by vacuum

rubber band
stretched around
base of chamber

Physicists hate to use the term "suction," but this time-honored method fills the penis with enough blood to make it firm. If the vacuum chamber were large enough to allow your partner to get inside, you would be all set. It appears to be more practical to slip a rubber band around the base of the penis to hold the blood in. This allows you to remove the chamber and have sex with a partner who is at standard atmospheric pressure. The band can be left on for about half an hour. The penis is firm only beyond the band, which means that the part attached to the body is soft, allowing a "hinge" action to occur. For this reason, the erection produced is not exactly the same as a natural one.

The advantages of this method are that it does not require injection, drugs, or surgery and cannot produce an emergency such as priapism. Its disadvantages are that it may occasionally cause bruising, that it lacks spontaneity, and that it can be somewhat cumbersome. As one of my patients put it, "you may not want to bring it on your first date."

Surgery

Over the years, effective technology has evolved to fill the interior of the erection chambers with some type of implanted cylinder and create an artificial erection. *Penile implant surgery* was for a time the only reliable way to restore erections in an impotent man. With the development of other effective alternatives, it has taken its place among a variety of options.

Although surgery is expensive and involves risks, it offers advantages that medical therapy does not. With successful implant surgery there is no need to carry around medical supplies or pneumatic devices, and the erection produced by an implant can be safely sustained for prolonged periods of time.

Two types of implants are currently in use: those with solid cylinders that can be bent down when off duty to avoid an obtrusive appearance, and those with inflatable cylinders. The second type is inflated by squeezing a bulb that is implanted in the scrotum or by squeezing a part of the cylinders that acts as a pump. The solid, bendable, *malleable implants* have the virtue of simplicity and fewer

FIGURE 8-9
Malleable Implant

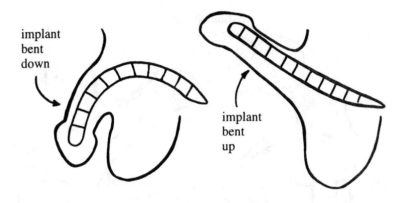

mechanical failures but create a permanent erection that either points up or down, depending upon your mood.

An *inflatable implant* with the pump in the scrotum creates the closest resemblance to a normal erection, in that it enlarges both in length and in diameter, then becomes reasonably flaccid when deflated. Its disadvantages are that the surgical procedure is more complicated, and the device has a higher chance of mechanical failure. With current technology, reliability is reasonably acceptable: there is approximately a 10 percent chance that some type of mechanical malfunction will occur in a six- to eight-year time span. Either type of implant can be placed during a short hospitalization—an outpatient visit or a single overnight stay in most cases.

The implant does not alter sensation, feeling, or climax—it just creates stiffness. While this may be what some patients are seeking, care should be exercised in making the decision to undergo surgery. Implant surgery will create a usable erection, but it may not correct problems that have developed within a relationship, or rectify other psychological issues that surface in sexual dysfunction. Deciding about surgery is best done after the patient and his partner have had an opportunity to discuss the situation with the doctor together.

FIGURE 8-10
Inflatable Implant

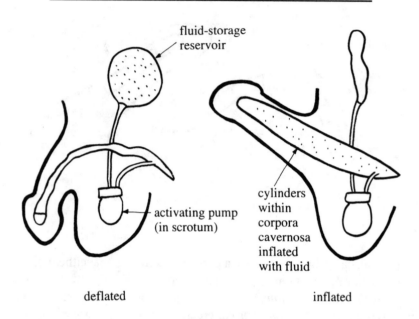

fluid-storage
reservoir

activating pump
(in scrotum)

cylinders
within
corpora
cavernosa
inflated
with fluid

deflated   inflated

Prostate problems don't always affect erections or sexual performance, but they do call attention to the parts of your anatomy that
may have worked more automatically in the past. Increased awareness of your own sexual responses can have a negative effect if it is
not mediated by increased understanding. Obtaining medical assistance is a good first step if things are not working well, but you'll
also need a positive attitude. Be willing to tolerate variation in the
degree of your desire and performance, as you get to know your own
natural rhythms. Increase communication with your partner—there
are more ways to entertain than you may have imagined.

Chapter 9

NUTRITION AND THE PROSTATE

The previous chapters have dealt exclusively with the biology of men's plumbing and conventional treatment for prostate disorders. Fortunately, keeping healthy is not as demanding a task as understanding illness and healing the sick. It is something we do naturally, with pleasure. In this chapter, we take a look at some naturally occurring food and plant products, and ways they have been used to promote men's health.

Science is a method for creating understanding and recognizing the order present in nature's patterns. Much of what is known about nutrition in health and disease is a product of the scientific method, although the medicinal use of naturally occurring substances predates the earliest laboratory science. While scientific understanding is mandatory for those treating disease, keeping healthy can safely proceed along guidelines set by tradition, native cultures, or your mother. There are few things more important than your own individual health, but society correctly recognizes that there is more risk in healing the sick than in maintaining the healthy. While we recognize the need for nutritional research, it makes sense that guidelines for healing are held to a higher standard of proof than ways to keep healthy.

All day long we are confronted by magazine articles and television doctors bombarding us with information. The dangers of too much or not enough cholesterol, the risk of fatty foods, the benefits of bran and fiber, the value of nutrition in preventing disease are all hot topics of discussion—for a good reason. There are things you can do right now that may decrease your chances of having prostate problems.

EATING WELL

Nutrition is the science that charts the relationships between what we eat and our health. An enormous range of vital bodily functions—from blood cell production to nerve conduction, bone strength, cardiac performance, reproduction, and emotional status—is affected by nutritional factors. These critical functions take place daily in people around the world who eat a wide variety of foods. While there are many at home and abroad who are too impoverished to receive adequate nutrition, the ability of a wide variety of dietary styles to maintain health in those fortunate enough to eat well is an important observation.

It is wise to avoid the faddish practices popularized by those who adhere to particularly rigid or special diets. Consider the wide range of diets that keep people healthy around the world—our relationship to the plants and animals we eat is as complex as we are. In addition to the guidelines below, recognizing the importance of dietary diversity is the first step toward good nutrition.

DIET AND THE PROSTATE

Nutritional factors complicate prostate problems in certain areas of the world. Bladder stones, rare in this country, occur commonly in parts of Southeast Asia, where vitamin B_6 deficiency is found. A lack of this essential vitamin increases the urinary excretion of oxylate, a substance that is prone to crystallize into stones. When oxylate concentrations in the urine are high, it doesn't take much stagnation of urine in the bladder from BPH before stones begin to form.

Studies have shown that prostate cancer is more common when a man's diet contains high amounts of animal fats and meats. Although one study found that large amounts of polyunsaturated fat (plant-derived fat that reduces blood cholesterol levels) increased the risk of cancer, animal fats from red meats were most closely linked to the risk of prostate cancer. Men who consumed the highest amounts of animal fat in one study were two and a half times as likely to die of prostate cancer, or be initially diagnosed with advanced prostate cancer, as those with low-fat diets. Several studies have shown that body weight and the risk of prostate cancer are related—the higher your percentage of body fat, the higher the risk. The protective effect of dietary fiber and vegetables in preventing colon cancer is fairly well established, but prostate cancer has not been studied as carefully in this regard. Indirect evidence from the study of blood hormone levels in women with breast cancer suggests a similar relationship. Like prostate cancer, breast cancer is a hormone-dependent tumor, and some studies have reported a reduction in blood hormone levels with high-fiber diets. This may suggest that fiber-rich foods could reduce the incidence of other hormone-dependent cancers.

In keeping with the general principles just mentioned, researchers have found that patients receive the greatest cancer prevention potential by consuming a wide variety of foods. In selecting the foods you eat, the National Cancer Institute has issued six recommendations, based on the findings of contemporary research:

1. At most, 30 percent of your calories should come from fat.
2. Fiber intake should be 20 to 30 grams per day—but no more than 35 grams. This means a fruit, vegetable, or grain serving with every meal.
3. Include a variety of vegetables and fruits in your diet.
4. Avoid obesity.
5. Moderate your alcohol consumption.
6. Minimize your consumption of smoked or salt-cured foods.

OTHER POSSIBILITIES

Professional nutritionists limit their general recommendations to opinions expressed in the "consensus documents" issued by the National Institutes of Health, the Surgeon General's office, and the National Cancer Institute. These guidelines are supported by well-conducted studies and accepted scientific laboratory research. They establish the basis for the broad, inclusive nutritional strategies but cannot extend to all possible nutritional factors or to therapeutic ideas originating in native or folk traditions.

Nutritional or herbal remedies for men with prostate problems are offered here. In contrast to treatments covered in other parts of this book, their scientific basis is scant or nonexistent. Although this limits the certainty with which specific recommendations can be made, it does not detract from the interest we all have in uncovering the potential benefits of folk healing.

The Pumpkin Seed

Herbalists say that nature produces a plant to combat every disease. If the prostate has such a plant it could be the pumpkin. The pulp of this well-known, plentiful member of the squash family is over-looked as a food source in favor of its once-a-year transformation into jack-o'-lanterns. Its seeds, which are salted, cooked, and packaged into nutritional worthlessness, are usually consumed only in baseball dugouts in this country.

Seeds are among the most complete foods known, because as single entities that must create new life, they must contain every element necessary for growth. Tapping into this wealth has long been advised by nutritional healers.

Pumpkin seeds (the raw, hulled ones only) have been a folk remedy against male impotence in Eastern European countries, where the rural folk eat them the way they eat sunflower seeds in Russia. It was not until the late 1920s, however, that research at the

University of Vienna revealed a lower incidence of BPH in these remote areas of the continent. The common dominator among the men surveyed: the pumpkin seed.

Pumpkin seeds contain large amounts of zinc, magnesium, and oleic acid, which appear to be important elements in keeping your prostate and sex life healthy.

Magnesium

Magnesium is a mineral found in the bones, essential to enzyme reactions in the metabolism of carbohydrates and in the stimulation of muscles and nerves. One of the things that age brings is magnesium deficiency. The lack of minimum amounts of this mineral may adversely affect both your prostate and your potency.

To keep this mineral at its proper level in the body is absolutely essential to good health. Foods rich in magnesium are peanuts, dried lima beans, corn, dried peas, soy flour, almonds, beet greens, Brazil nuts, cashews, endive, hazelnuts, and walnuts. And don't forget the pumpkin seed.

Zinc

Trace minerals are elements needed in minuscule amounts by the body. Deficiency can lead to serious disturbances in the functioning of the body's organs and glands. When it comes to the prostate, one of the most important trace minerals is zinc. Large amounts of zinc are stored in the prostate, and there is a relationship between disease and a deficiency of zinc. Studies have shown that there are lower levels of zinc in prostates with malignant tumors. Whether this is cause or effect is unknown.

Semen is also extremely rich in zinc, although the testis is relatively poor in this mineral. It is likely that the prostate supplies and holds zinc-containing fluids until ejaculation. Zinc appears to be a necessary element for both prostate health and potency.

Foods rich in zinc are onions, eggs, molasses, beef liver, rabbit, chicken, rice bran, gelatin, lentils, nuts, and brewer's yeast.

Lecithin

This compound may be a factor in prostate health. *Lecithin* is a fatty substance that occurs in the cellular tissues of living things. The polyunsaturated fats in lecithin cause the breakdown of the cholesterol portion of fat and prevent its accumulation on the blood vessel walls. In one nutritional study, men with enlarged prostates who were given doses of unsaturated fatty acids showed reduction of residual urine, less need to get up at night to urinate, increased sexual drive, less dribbling, increased force of the urinary stream, and reduction in the size of the prostate.

Lecithin comes from the Greek *lekithos,* which is the name for the yolk of an egg, so naturally they are a recommended food. Other foods rich in lecithin are melon seeds, nuts, wheat germ, brains, safflower oil, corn oil, soybean oil, liver, beef, barley seeds, corn seeds, sunflower seeds, and of course pumpkin seeds.

Amino Acids

Amino acids, the basic building blocks of protein, are found in all living things and therefore exist naturally in food. Their effectiveness in treating prostatitis was discovered by accident when two doctors were treating a group of patients suffering from allergies with a mixture of three amino acids (glycine, alanine, and glutamic acid). One of their patients mentioned that his long-standing urinary problems had disappeared, and the hunt was on. Other patients with urinary problems were treated with amino therapy, and the majority reported prompt and spectacular relief as long as they took the amino mixture.

Food rich in these three amino acids are beef, calves', and chicken liver; lean beef, lamb, and veal; brewer's yeast, nonfat dry milk; eggs and egg yolks; kidney beans, lentils, peanuts, and soybeans; corn and whole wheat flour.

A diet low in fat and high in complex carbohydrates is routinely prescribed by nutritionists everywhere as a general health recommendation and would certainly be wise for those with difficulties caused by a swollen prostate gland. A diet high in amino acids may not be easily handled by persons with reduced kidney function, however.

Herbs

Human beings have discovered, by trial and error, which plants and herbs might be used for food or for medicinal purposes. Folk medicine, consisting of the use of these selected plants, originated out of necessity and still exists. The Chinese, for example, have a comprehensive herbal manual, with over one thousand ancient herbal remedies, that is still authoritative. Every part of the human body is covered, the prostate included. Herbal treatments, while they do offer comfort and relief, are no substitute for professional medical care. Some popular herbal remedies for the prostate are these:

1. Enlargement or inflammation of the prostate has been treated by drinking herbal teas.
2. A mixture of hydrangea root, holly, and gravel root has also been used to ease inflammation and urinary burning.
3. Other herbs thought to be effective for prostate problems are parsley, juniper berries, slippery elm bark, goldenseal root, *Serenoa serrulata (Saw Palmetto)* and *Pygeum africanum.*
4. For male reproductive problems a tonic of ginseng root is often used.

In conclusion, try to incorporate variety and some of the accepted nutritional guidelines into your diet. If you are having urinary or sexual difficulties, see your doctor. Even if you have no problems, you should have a yearly PSA test and a prostate examination if you are over fifty. When medical evaluation fails to show serious problems behind bothersome symptoms, you may find benefit from the natural products just described.

Chapter 10

AGING IS A DISEASE—AND OTHER MISCONCEPTIONS

This book was written to dispel the fear that comes from not knowing the truth about the prostate and its problems. In addition to creating apprehension, ignorance is a fertile source of misunderstanding. Some of these misplaced beliefs are amusing, and a few of them are dangerous. They have a way of combining with each other and compounding into larger perspectives that gradually distort one's overall outlook. Unraveling these misconceptions will help us recap much of the material in the preceding chapters.

Only old men have a prostate. All males are born with a prostate gland, and it follows a certain pattern of growth and change during life. Of course, problems arising from the prostate are more common later in life.

The prostate gland sits inside the rectum. The prostate gland is part of the urinary tract, outside the rectum but next to it.

Sperm are squeezed out of the testicles during ejaculation. Sperm are made in the testicles but stored in the ampullary, or dilated ends of the vas deferens. Contraction of this tubing pushes the sperm into the urethra during ejaculation.

Only teenagers have hormones. Adults have them, too—they are just tired. Hormones are an internal chemical control system that all people have. Their effects are most noticeable during puberty, when the bodily alterations that occur are the result of their activity.

Trouble with urinating means prostate problems. There are a variety of causes for most urinary symptoms. For example, slowing of the stream does not mean prostate cancer is present.

Frequent urination is due to weak kidneys. Frequent urination is almost always due to malfunction of the bladder, not the kidneys.

Prostate problems cause insomnia. They may cause increased nighttime urination, but they don't cause sleep disorders. If the problem is severe enough, however, you can lose a lot of sleep getting up to visit the bathroom eight or ten times a night.

Dribbling after urination means prostate cancer. This nuisance is common and does not mean cancer is present.

Serious urinary blockage of the bladder by the prostate always produces bothersome symptoms. This is usually true, but occasionally damaging blockage can occur with minimal or no symptoms.

Blood in the urine means cancer. The most common cause of blood in the urine in men over fifty is *benign* prostatic hypertrophy (BPH). Although it usually is not a sign of cancer, all cases of blood in the urine should be checked by a doctor.

Prostate rectal examination causes sexual stimulation. Although the anal area can be an erogenous zone, this is not true. Virtually all patients feel the exam is moderately uncomfortable, and they are glad that it takes much less than a minute to do.

Blood tests reveal most diseases. In general, most diagnoses can be made from symptoms and examination. In the case of the PSA test, abnormalities do not always indicate prostate cancer.

Prostatitis is always caused by bacteria. Inflammation of the prostate, or prostatitis, is not always the result of infection with bacteria or other microorganisms.

Prostatitis is caused by too much sex. Overindulgence may make you sore, but it does not usually contribute to this condition.

Prostatitis is caused by too little sex. Congestion, or buildup of semen in the prostate, can cause some of the symptoms of prostatitis.

Urinary infections are common and a fever means the body is fighting it off. Urinary infections in men are not common and should prompt medical evaluation. When a urinary tract infection is accompanied by fever, it is particularly dangerous and should warrant immediate medical attention.

BPH is caused by increasing hormone levels in older men. Actually, the level of the male sex hormone, testosterone, decreases slightly with age.

BPH can be prevented by frequent ejaculations. This condition is not caused by sexual inactivity.

Symptoms of BPH mean you will need surgery some day. Most men with symptoms due to BPH do not end up having surgery.

New medications have eliminated the need for prostate surgery. Medications have reduced the need for surgery in benign enlargement, but there are still conditions that require operations: catheter dependency and bladder stones, for example.

Antihistamines and other cold remedies cause the prostate to swell. While it is true that these medications should not be used in men with symptomatic BPH, they do not cause the prostate to swell. Rather, they constrict the muscle fibers around the urethra and weaken the muscular contraction of the bladder wall.

Bladder stones are caused by too much salt. Most bladder stones form when there is obstruction and "stagnation" of urine. They also form in men with gout, when there is too much uric acid in the urine. In some parts of the world, bladder stones can be the result of vitamin B_6 deficiency.

BPH surgery can always be postponed, as the effects of this disorder are reversible. In cases of severe blockage, the bladder wall can be irreversibly damaged, making it difficult to urinate even after the obstruction has been relieved surgically. In these cases, surgery can be safely postponed for weeks, but not for years.

Bothersome symptoms of BPH are unheard of before age sixty-five. Symptoms of BPH become more common with age, but studies have shown that 12 to 15 percent of men in their forties and fifties are bothered by a slow stream, urgency, and the need to get up frequently at night to urinate.

I had my prostate removed, so I can't get cancer. Operations for BPH are called "removing the prostate," but this is somewhat misleading. Surgical treatment of BPH consists of removing the overgrown transitional zone in the middle of the prostate, leaving a shell of peripheral zone prostate tissue. This remaining prostate can be a source of prostate cancer in the years that follow.

Surgery for BPH makes you impotent. A TURP or an open prostatectomy will reduce or eliminate the discharge of semen with orgasm, but it rarely alters erection in someone who was sexually active prior to surgery.

Surgery for BPH leads to cancer. Before the days of PSA tests, occult or previously undetected cancer was found in up to 10 percent of the prostates "removed" for BPH. In this sense, surgery leads to the diagnosis of cancer. Surgery for BPH does not cause cancer or increase your chances of subsequently developing it.

I can't have prostate cancer—I have no symptoms. Curable prostate cancer usually produces no symptoms.

I am going to die of my prostate cancer—it is an incurable disease. Most men with prostate cancer don't die of it. When it is treated early, the disease-free survival times of men who have had prostate cancer is about the same as the life expectancy of men of the same age without prostate cancer.

Prostate cancer is so slow-growing that treatment is unnecessary. While this may be true in older men with early cancer, men with a life expectancy of ten years or more, or those with symptoms due to spreading cancer, should be treated. Early prostate cancer in younger men should always be treated aggressively, as it will inevitably progress, given enough time.

After treatment for prostate cancer I will have to live my life differently. Some adjustments may be necessary, but most men return to their usual routine after treatment.

Impotence is an inevitable consequence of aging. As men get older, erections may become fewer in number and more difficult to obtain, but they should not disappear. Most research points to physical causes, not just "getting older."

Prostate problems herald the onset of impotence. Both of these medical problems are increasingly more common with age, but prostate disorders don't as a rule cause problems with erection.

Impotence is a psychosomatic problem. Most cases of erectile dysfunction have a physical cause—the problem is not usually psychological. However, psychological reactions to change in potency are often significant, and it would be wrong to say that psychologic factors don't play a role.

Penile implant surgery will restore your sex life. This operation will make the penis stiff. Depending on it to resolve marital conflicts or find you a new girlfriend may be asking too much.

Men with prostate problems should wait until the bladder is full to obtain a better, longer-lasting erection. Erections occur as a reflex when the bladder fills up, but this practice can lead to urinary difficulty in men with blockage due to BPH.

Masturbation leads to impotence. This is a version of the "you-have-only-a-limited-amount-of-orgasms-in-you" theory, which is not true.

After vasectomy, ejaculation does not occur. There is still ejaculation of fluid, in the usual amount, after vasectomy. The semen no longer contain sperm cells, however.

Eating a proper diet will prevent cancer. Some scientifically valid studies have shown that dietary makeup affects the incidence of certain cancers in some groups of people. While adjusting your eating habits to conform with these findings certainly makes sense, there is no proof of this statement in general.

Prostate enlargement can be reduced by eating pumpkin seeds. The background for this belief lies in anecdotal "reports," not controlled scientific studies.

Vegetarians perform better in bed. Maybe in a bed of lettuce . . . seriously, there is no support for this belief.

If a nutrient is essential in small quantities, more is better. This belief is responsible for megavitamin "therapy." Ask any gardener—citrus trees need trace amounts of iron, but they can't be raised in a barrel full of nails.

Eating animal fats causes impotence. Indirectly, a diet high in animal fats may (if other factors are present) contribute to arterial disease that could affect erections. There is no direct connection, however.

Zinc will cure most prostate problems. The prostate contains high concentrations of zinc, but a therapeutic effect from taking zinc has never been proved.

High-fiber diets prolong erection. Dietary fiber is good for you, but there is nothing to support this idea.

Aging is a disease. Life is continuous change, and the physical alterations that occur from middle life onward can be a nuisance. You don't have to look far before coming across euphemisms such as "the golden years" or others coined by people selling retirement property. This chirpy sales pitch misstates the process of aging, but not as badly as the concept that growing older is some type of disorder. Years give us aches, pains, and doctor visits but also the wisdom to understand and accept the trade-offs. It would be nice to combine the experience and perspective of age with the physical vigor of youth, when the body spins onward through every day with scarcely a notice. The closest we can come to this is when we are surrounded by a family or community that spans many age groups and fosters contact among all generations. When elders are included in this way, they have their own unique power. In this setting, living long becomes neither disease nor exaltation, but simply the way of life in human form.

The ultimate goal of medicine is immortality. Doctors must offer their patients ways to stay healthy and options to restore health when disease occurs. We need to do our best to communicate what we know to the patient and to listen to what the patient tells us. As physicians, we are morally compelled to offer treatment for every situation, but patient and doctor alike know that in certain situations life must come to an end. Physicians do not have to view death as the enemy in every encounter in order to hold life in the highest regard or to practice compassionate healing. Prostate cancer is not always fatal, but we might do well to ponder the question of an ancient Chinese philosopher, Chuang Tzu: How do I know that in hating death I am not like a man who, having left home in his youth, has forgotten the way back?

GLOSSARY

Adenoma A benign tumor that originates in a gland.

Alpha-adrenergic receptors Neuromuscular control sites present in muscle surrounding the urethra, causing contraction when activated.

Alpha blockers Drugs that block alpha receptors and prevent them from causing muscle contraction.

Amino acids The constituent building blocks of proteins.

Aminoglutethimide A drug that inhibits function of the adrenal gland.

Aneuploid A cell having abnormal amounts of DNA.

Angiography X-ray study of blood vessels, made by injecting dye (contrast material).

Anterior superior iliac spines The forwardmost and highest corners of the pelvis, which can be felt under the skin of the lower abdomen.

Apex The lowest point of the prostate (the end that faces the penis, not the bladder).

Atonic Having complete lack of muscle contraction.

Autologous blood donation Use of a patient's own banked blood for transfusion.

Azoospermia Complete absence of sperm in the semen.

Bacteremia Bacteria present in the bloodstream.

Bacterial prostatitis Prostate infection due to bacteria.

Benign prostatic hypertrophy (BPH) Noncancerous enlargement of the prostate.

Biopsy Removal of a piece of tissue for diagnostic purposes.

Bladder diverticulum Outpouching or "blowout" of the bladder, usually due to obstruction.

Bladder neck Lowermost part, or "outlet," of the bladder.

Bladder spasm Painful cramping of the bladder, usually caused by bladder surgery.

Blood urea nitrogen (BUN) A measure of nitrogen-containing waste products in the blood, used to gauge kidney function.

Cancer A disease characterized by abnormalities of cellular growth control that are passed on to each new generation of cells.

Carbenicillin Antibiotic used for prostatitis.

Catheter Tube used to drain urine from bladder.

Cavernous nerves Nerves controlling erectile function.

Cell membrane The outer wall of a cell.

Central zone One of the inner parts of the prostate, surrounds the entrance of the ejaculatory ducts into the urethra.

Cephalexin Broad-spectrum antibiotic.

Chemotherapy Use of cytotoxic (cell-poisoning) medications to treat cancer.

Chlamydia Microorganism that can cause urethritis and epididymitis.

Chromosomes Sites within cell nucleus where genetic material is stored.

Ciprofloxacin Antibiotic used in urinary tract infections.

Clinical staging Determination of the anatomical extent of cancer by use of tests, not surgery.

Clot retention Inability to urinate when blood clots block the bladder.

Collagen Protein that serves as the body's chief structural or strength-producing element.

Compensated obstruction In the bladder, overcoming of blockage by increasing force of muscular contraction.

Contact inhibition Property exhibited by noncancerous cells growing in culture, where cell division is inhibited by crowding.

Contrast agents X-ray dyes.

Corpora cavernosa The paired cylindrical chambers within the penis that expand with blood during erection.

Creatinine clearance A measure of the kidney's excretory function.

Cryotherapy Freezing the prostate to treat cancer.

Cyproterone acetate Medication that blocks the effects of testosterone on cells.

Cystoscope Endoscope used to view the interior of the urethra, prostate, and bladder.

Deoxyribonucleic acid (DNA) The genetic material of all cells. It is a long molecule, whose makeup encodes the information necessary for the assembly of proteins.

Dialysis Treatment used to remove wastes from the bloodstream, when the kidneys have failed.

Diazepam Muscle relaxant and antianxiety drug.

Diethystilbestrol An oral form of estrogen (female hormone).

Dihydrotestosterone The activated form of testosterone, which is responsible for most of its effects within the cell.

Diploid The normal amount of DNA present in cells (one pair of each chromosome).

Directed donation The donation of blood for a designated recipient.

Distensibility The ability to expand freely without having to stretch too tightly.

Diuretics Drugs that increase urine output.

Double voiding Needing to urinate a short time after voiding.

Doxycycline Antibiotic used to treat prostatitis, urethritis, and epididymitis.

Drain Plastic or rubber tube used to allow fluids to escape from the site of surgery.

Dynamic obstruction Bladder blockage caused by contraction of muscles around the urethra.

Ejaculation Forceful expulsion of semen.

Ejaculatory ducts The tubes that channel fluids from the converging vas deferens and the seminal vesicles into the prostatic urethra during ejaculation.

Endocrine glands Glands that secrete substances into the bloodstream.

Endoscopy Looking into the body with special optical equipment.

Enuresis Nighttime urinary leakage, bedwetting.

Enzyme Protein that serves as a catalyst for (increases the rate of) chemical reactions.

Epididymis Duct that channels sperm from the testis to the vas deferens.

Epididymitis Painful disorder caused by inflammation of the epididymis.

Erectile dysfunction Difficulty obtaining or maintaining a hard erection.

Erythromycin Antibiotic used for urethritis and prostatitis.

Estrogen Female sex hormone.

Exocrine glands Glands that excrete substances into specially formed duct systems.

Extraperitoneal Outside the peritoneal (intestinal) cavity.

Finasteride Drug that blocks the conversion of testosterone to dihydrotestosterone.

Flutamide Drug that blocks the effect of testosterone on cells; used against prostate cancer.

Foley Self-retaining urinary catheter, held in by a small balloon that inflates within the bladder.

Frozen section technique Method for rapidly processing biopsy samples; allows pathologist to make microscopic diagnosis during the course of surgery.

Gamma-seminoprotein Protein present in semen; the measure of its level in blood is known as the prostate-specific antigen (PSA) level.

Genes The factors present in organisms that transmit hereditary traits to offspring; known to be segments of the DNA molecule.

Gleason system Scale for grading the microscopic abnormalities in prostate cancer.

Glomerulus Microscopic filtration unit in the kidney.

Goserelin acetate Medication that reduces testosterone output by diminishing the pituitary gland's output of a regulatory chemical.

Grade The degree of cellular abnormality in a cancer.

Hematospermia Blood in the semen.

Histologic cancer Cancer incidentally discovered in the prostate at autopsy, that was not diagnosed during life.

Hormone deprivation Treatment of prostate cancer by lowering the blood testosterone level.

Hydronephrosis Dilation or ''ballooning'' of the kidney due to blockage.

Hypertrophied Increased in size.

Hypoechoic Producing less echo signal on an ultrasound; showing as a dark area.

Hytrin® Alpha blocker drug used to treat BPH.

Iliac crest Upper rim of the pelvic bone.

Implants Rods or cylinders surgically placed inside the corpora cavernosa to restore erection.

Impotence Inability to get or keep an erection hard enough for intercourse.

Incontinence Involuntary urinary leakage.

Infarction Tissue death due to lack of blood supply.

Infertility Inability to conceive a pregnancy.

Inflammation The biological response to injury or infection, that leads into the processes of healing and tissue repair.

Intravenous pyelogram (IVP) An X-ray study of the kidneys, ureters, and bladder, obtained by the intravenous administration of X-ray dye.

Laparoscope Endoscope used to work within the abdominal cavity.

Laparoscopic lymphadenectomy Diagnostic operation using laparoscope to remove lymph nodes.

Laser prostatectomy Incision or ablation (destruction) of obstructing prostate tissue using laser light.

Lateral lobe enlargement Pattern of BPH in which a pair of tissue masses sit side by side, compressing the urethra between them.

Leuprolide Medication that reduces testosterone output by inhibiting the pituitary gland's production of a regulatory chemical.

Leydig cells Cells within the testicle that make testosterone.

Libido Sex drive or desire.

Lomefloxacin Antibiotic used in urinary tract infections.

Luteinizing hormone Messenger hormone made by the pituitary gland that affects testosterone secretion by the testicle.

Luteinizing hormone releasing factor Messenger chemical secreted by the brain, which controls release of luteinizing hormone from the pituitary gland.

Lymphadenectomy Surgical removal of lymph nodes.

Malignant transformation Conversion of normal cells into cancer cells.

Margins The edges of a specimen removed from the body at surgery.

Median lobe hypertrophy Pattern of BPH in which enlargement occurs in one single mass of tissue that sits in the center of the bladder neck.

Metastases Secondary deposits caused by spread of cancer.

Minipress® Alpha blocker used to treat BPH.

Minocycline Antibiotic used to treat urethritis, prostatitis, and epididymitis.

Myogenic Originating in muscle.

Nephron Tiny tube that is the filtration and fluid-processing element within the kidney.

Neurotransmitters Chemicals that transmit nerve signals.

Neurogenic bladder A bladder that fills or contracts abnormally because of a disorder of its nerves.

Nitric oxide The neurotransmitter chemical that is responsible for the erection initiated by cavernous nerve signals.

Nocturnal tumescence Nighttime erections.

Norfloxacin Antibiotic used for urinary tract infections.

Nucleus Central part of cell, containing chromosomes.

Oncogenes DNA segments (genes) that can play a role in the malignant transformation of cells.

Open prostatectomy Operation for removal of obstruction due to BPH, performed through incision in the skin.

Orchiectomy Removal of testicle(s).

Ofloxacin Antibiotic used for urinary tract infections.

Overflow incontinence Leakage due to a bladder that can't empty.

Palliative Treatment offered for purposes of improvement rather than for cure.

Papaverine Medication used to treat impotence.

Pathologist Physician specializing in the effects of disease on tissue; responsible for biopsy interpretation.

Penile-brachial index The ratio of blood pressure in the arm to that in the penis, used to diagnose blood vessel disease as the cause of impotence.

Perineum The area between the anus and the scrotum.

Peripheral zone The outer part of the prostate, where most cancers form.

Peritoneal cavity Body cavity that contains the abdominal viscera.

Placebo Inactive substance used in drug testing to separate psychologic effects from drug activity.

Ploidy Refers to the DNA content of cells.

Ports Areas of the body where radiation enters during therapy.

Prazosin Alpha blocker medication used to treat BPH.

Proscar® Drug that blocks the activation of testosterone, used to treat BPH.

Prostaglandins Compounds forming a part of the body's system of internal chemical controls; also a medication used in the treatment of impotence.

Prostate-specific antigen (PSA) Test for gamma-seminoprotein in the bloodstream, used to detect and monitor prostate cancer.

Prostatic fossa Open space within the prostate, following TURP or open prostatectomy.

Prostatic urethra The part of the urinary channel, or urethra, that passes through the prostate.

Prostatism Symptoms of urinary tract obstruction due to prostate enlargement.

Prostatitis Inflammation of the prostate.

Prostatodynia Painful prostate.

Refractory period Period of time following climax and loss of erection, when it is impossible to obtain a second erection.

Remission Response of cancer to therapy.

Resectoscope Endoscopic instrument used to resect, or remove, inner portions of the prostate during TURP.

Residual urine Urine remaining in the bladder after voiding.

Retrograde ejaculation During climax, exit of semen from the prostatic urethra into the bladder, rather than out the end of the penis.

Seminal vesicles Sac-like chambers attached to the prostate, that lie behind the bladder and secrete fluids into semen.

Sepsis Illness caused by bacteremia.

Serum creatinine Blood test used to monitor the kidney's filtering effectiveness.

Silent prostatism Urinary tract blockage due to BPH that occurs without symptoms.

Sinusoids Microscopic muscle-walled chambers in the penis that fill with blood during erection.

Stage The anatomical extent of a cancer.

Static obstruction Blockage of bladder due to compression and distortion on the urethra by BPH.

Stroma Connective tissue that surrounds and supports glands within the prostate.

Suprapubic prostatectomy Open prostatectomy done through an incision in the bladder.

Suprapubic tube Urinary catheter that enters the bladder directly through the lower abdomen, without passing through the urethra.

Suprapubic prostatectomy Open prostatectomy done through an incision in the bladder.

Suprapubic tube Urinary catheter that enters the bladder directly through the lower abdomen, without passing through the urethra.

Suramin Investigational drug for use in advanced prostate cancer.

Surgical capsule The compressed shell of outer prostate that forms as BPH enlarges within.

Terazosin Alpha blocker drug used to treat BPH.

Testosterone Male sex hormone.

Tetracycline Antibiotic used to treat prostatitis and urethritis.

Trabeculation Irregular, webbed configuration of the bladder that occurs in response to obstruction.

Transition zone Inner part of the prostate, where BPH forms.

Transurethral incision of the prostate (TUIP) Operation for obstruction due to BPH, involving incisions in the bladder neck.

Transurethral resection of the prostate (TURP) Operation for blockage due to BPH, involving endoscopic removal of obstructing tissue.

Trilobar hypertrophy Pattern of BPH involving both lateral lobe and median lobe enlargement.

Trimethoprim-sulfa Antibiotic used for prostatitis and other urinary tract infections.

True capsule Thin connective tissue layer forming the border around the prostate gland.

Tumor suppressor genes DNA segments that inhibit cell growth and can contribute to cancer when blocked or suppressed.

Tumoricidal Tumor-killing.

Tunica albuginea Strong covering layer of the corpora cavernosa that contributes to penile rigidity during erection.

Ultrasound The use of high-frequency sound waves to create anatomical images of the body.

Ureter Muscular tube that conducts urine from the kidney into the bladder.

Urethra The urinary channel that conducts urine out of the bladder.

Urethral stricture Scar that narrows the urethra.

Urinary flow rate Measurement of the speed of urinary flow.

Urinary retention Inability to urinate.

Urodynamic testing Measurement of fluid pressure and flow characteristics to diagnose urinary tract malfunction.

Vacuum erection devices Devices used to increase the hardness of an erection, by filling the penis with blood by externally applied vacuum.

Vas deferens The tube that conducts sperm from the testis and epididymis to the prostatic urethra.

Verumontanum Entry site in the prostatic urethra of the ejaculatory ducts.

Yohimbe Bark extract used to treat impotence.

Yohimbine hydrochloride Purified active ingredient of yohimbe, used as a prescription medication to treat impotence.

INDEX

Page numbers in *italics* refer to illustrations.

progression of, 140–41, 142–43,
142, 149, 150, 157, 158, 160–61,
230
after prostate removal, 15, 84, 229
PSA test and, 24, 44, 100, 115–16,
131–32, 133–34, 135, 137, 138
race and geography in, 117–18
rectal exam and, 40–41, 100, 131,
133, 134, 155, 157
remission of, 161, 242
screening for, 134–35
seminal vesicles affected by, 158,
159
sexual desire and, 38
size of, 143
staging in, 137–40, 148, 155–63,
187–88, 189
statistics on, 117–18
symptoms of, 125–27
systemic, 143
ultrasound and, 52–54, 127, 133
vasectomy and, 118
zinc and, 223
see also cancer
prostate cancer treatment, 119, 122,
140–63
for advanced cancer, 150–55
chemotherapy, 153, 155, 234
experimental, 150
hormone deprivation, *see* hormone
deprivation treatment
for localized cancer, 143, 144
making decisions about, 141–43, 144
progression of disease with no treatment, 140–41
quality-of-life issues in, 149–50, 162
radiation, *see* radiation therapy
results and recommendations for, 150,
155–63
in stage A, 155–58
in stage B, 156, 158–59
in stage C, 156, 159–60
in stage D, 156, 160–63
surgery, 164, 170–71, 187–92; *see
also* prostate surgery
watchful waiting and, 144, 149–50,
152, 156
prostate gland, 9–27, 199, 202, 226
abscess in, 65, *67*
central zone of, 14, *15,* 234

congestion in, 228
definition and function of, 9, 10, 11–
12, 13
enlargement of, 9, 81, 115, 231; *see
also* benign prostatic hypertrophy;
urinary tract obstruction from
examination of fluid from, 43
formation of, 13–16, *14,* 29, 88
growth of, 24–27
hormones and, 104, 105–8
location of, 10–13, *10*
misconceptions about, 226–32
nerve control in, 22–23
nutrition and, *see* nutrition
peripheral zone of, 14, 15, *15,* 40, 53,
84, 125, 178, 229, 241
secretions of, 13, 16, 21–24, 69
sexual function and, 196, 204–10
stones in, 68, *68,* 70
surgical capsule of, 84, *84,* 179, 243
transition zone of, 14, 15, *15, 16,* 82,
83–84, 125, 171, 178, 229, 243
true capsule of, 84, *84,* 243
zones of, 14, 15, *15,* 53
prostate-specific antigen (PSA) test, 24,
44, 100, 101, 108, 115–16, 131–
135, 136, 137, 138, 141, 142, 148,
149, 157, 188, 206, 225, 227, 229,
241
age and, 131, 132
prostate surgery (prostatectomy), 15, 56,
77, 101, 143, 149, 157, 164–93,
228, 229
anesthesia for, 165–67
balloon dilation, 73, 113, 185, 191
blood transfusions and, 169–70, 172
for BPH and obstruction, 80–81, 86,
102, 103–4, 171–87
for cancer, 164, 170–71, 187–92
for chronic bacterial prostatitis, 68, 70
complications of, 172–73
drains and tubes used in, 167–68, *169,*
192, 236; *see also* catheters
endoscopic, *see* endoscopic surgery
intraurethral stents, 186
laser, 103–4, 183–85, 239
lower abdominal incision for, *178*
nerve-sparing, 208
open (simple), 113, 165, 171, 172,
177–81, *179,* 188–89, 229, 240

ABOUT THE AUTHORS

Martin K. Gelbard, M.D.

Dr. Martin Gelbard is a board-certified urologic surgeon with a private practice in Burbank, California. He is a clinical assistant professor of urology at the UCLA School of Medicine and an attending urologist at the Sepulveda Veterans Administration Hospital. He has written twenty-four scientific articles and four chapters in medical texts. Dr. Gelbard is a recognized contributor to the field of urologic reconstructive surgery and has been the recipient of two essay awards for original medical research. He is the author and principal investigator of three FDA-sanctioned clinical trials.

William Bentley

William Bentley is a Los Angeles–based screen and television writer. This is his first book.